Workbook
Laboratory
Testing
for Ambulatory
Settings

A Guide for Health Care Professionals

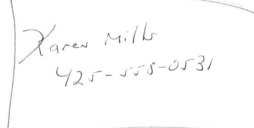

Marti Garrels, MSA, MT (ASCP), CMA
Professor and Program Chair
Medical Assisting Program
Ivy Tech Community College of Indiana
South Bend, Indiana

Carol Oatis, MSEd, MT SM (ASCP), CMA
Program Chair
Medical Assisting Program
Ivy Tech Community College of Indiana
Evansville, Indiana

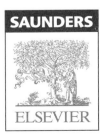

SAUNDERS

ELSEVIER

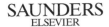

SAUNDERS
ELSEVIER

11830 Westline Industrial Drive
St. Louis, Missouri 63146

WORKBOOK FOR LABORATORY TESTING FOR AMBULATORY
SETTINGS: A GUIDE FOR HEALTH CARE PROFESSIONALS
Copyright © 2006 by Saunders, an imprint of Elsevier Inc.

ISBN-13: 978-0-7216-4787-6
ISBN-10: 0-7216-4787-1

Notice

Knowledge and best practice in this field are constantly changing. As new research and experience
broaden our knowledge, changes in practice, treatment and drug therapy may become necessary
or appropriate. Readers are advised to check the most current information provided (i) on
procedures featured or (ii) by the manufacturer of each product to be administered, to verify the
recommended dose or formula, the method and duration of administration, and contraindications.
It is the responsibility of the practitioner, relying on their own experience and knowledge of the
patient, to make diagnoses, to determine dosages and the best treatment for each individual
patient, and to take all appropriate safety precautions. To the fullest extent of the law, neither
the Publisher nor the Authors assume any liability for any injury and/or damage to persons or
property arising out or related to any use of the material contained in this book.

The Publisher

ISBN-13: 978-0-7216-4787-6
ISBN-10: 0-7216-4787-1

Publisher: Michael Ledbetter
Associate Developmental Editor: Katherine Judge
Publishing Services Manager: Pat Joiner
Project Manager: David Stein
Design Direction: Andrea Lutes

Working together to grow
libraries in developing countries

www.elsevier.com | www.bookaid.org | www.sabre.org

ELSEVIER | BOOK AID International | Sabre Foundation

Printed in the United States of America

Last digit is the print number: 9 8 7 6 5 4 3

Contents

Introduction

This workbook is designed to build mastery over the highly technical and fascinating field of laboratory medicine. Each chapter is organized into five sections: terminology exercises, review questions from basic concepts, procedures, advanced concepts, and check-off procedure sheets for all the procedures presented in the textbook chapter. The completed workbook exercises and check-off procedure sheets fulfill all the competency objectives listed at the beginning of each chapter in the textbook. The appendix of the workbook contains lab maintenance logs, report forms, quality control logs, patient logs, and a sample health screening assessment form. These forms provide the necessary documentation needed to prove laboratory quality assurance, safety compliance, and proper charting of test results.

Tips For Mastering Each Chapter

Terminology Exercises

Prior to reading each chapter, you should become familiar with the technical terms related to the subject. The CD, located in the text, provides tutorial exercises using the terms, and the matching exercises in this workbook will be very helpful for learning the terms. It is also recommended that you make flash cards of the terms. Then, as you read the text and fill in your structured notes (from the CD), you will find each of the terms bolded and defined in context to reinforce and build further understanding.

Basic Concepts, Procedures, Advanced Concepts—Review Questions and Labeling

The questions, pictures, and diagrams in these three sections fulfill the stated objectives for each chapter. The questions are designed to follow the textbook and structured notes from the CD. You are encouraged to use the textbook alongside the workbook for visual reinforcement and as a reference for finding data from the tables and flow charts. The advanced concepts sections contain more complex critical-thinking exercises, as well as referencing detailed laboratory test information in chapters 4 through 7. Your course instructor may assign one or more of these three sections, depending on the time frame of the course.

Check-off Procedure Sheets

These outcome-based procedure sheets are found at the end of each chapter. You are encouraged to locate in the textbook the corresponding procedure box, which provides pictures of the various steps involved in each procedure. The procedures fall into two categories: *Skill Procedures* (such as using a microscope, instructing patients, collecting specimens, and staining slides) and *Analytical Tests* in which you follow a test procedure in order to obtain test results (such as urinalysis, hemoglobin, glucose, and strep test). In both cases, it is very important that you read, perform, and check off each step on the sheet as satisfactory or unsatisfactory. The steps marked with an asterisk (✳) are critical to demonstrate competency. The *Skill Procedures* will generally be performed with the instructor verifying each step. The *Analytical Tests* may be performed with a lab partner verifying the steps leading up to the test result. The instructor would then verify the final test result and the proper documentation of the test result in order to fulfill the required measurable outcome.

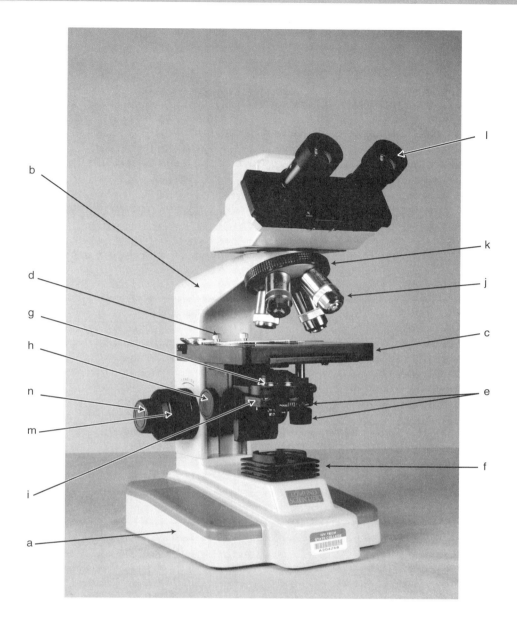

ADVANCED CONCEPTS

CLIA Government Regulations

____ 55. Tests that produce a result measured as a number

A. package insert

____ 56. A substance or ingredient used in a laboratory test to detect, measure, examine, or produce a reaction

B. quality assurance

____ 57. An *overall* process to aid in improving the reliability, efficiency, and quality of laboratory test results

C. qualitative

____ 58. Materials with known values of the substance measured that help the laboratory achieve accurate and reliable testing by checking if the test system is working

D. quality control

____ 59. Instructions included by the manufacturer located in the kit or test package

E. kit

_____ 60. Proving competency by testing a specimen from an outside accreditation agency

_____ 61. Tests that simply look for the presence or absence of a substance

_____ 62. A process in which known samples (controls) are routinely tested to establish the reliability, accuracy, and precision of a specific test system

_____ 63. All components of a test that are packaged together

F. quantitative

G. reagent

H. proficiency testing

I. controls

64. What is the purpose of the Clinical Laboratory Improvement Amendment (CLIA1988) and how does it benefit the patient?

_____

_____

65. What are the three categories of testing under CLIA, and under which category is physician-performed microscopy listed?

_____

_____

_____

66. Review Table 1-6 in the text, which lists most of the CLIA waived tests available. Locate three tests in each category and list their corresponding procedure codes below.

Test Category	Physician Office Tests	Procedure Code (CPT; 5-digit code)
Hematology tests		
Blood chemistry tests		
Serology/immunology tests		
Microbiology tests (only two)		

67. From the provider-performed microscopy procedure Table 1-7 in the text, write the procedure codes for each of the following:

a. Wet mounts, including preparations of vaginal, cervical, or skin specimens _____

b. Urinalysis (microscopic only)_____

c. All potassium hydroxide preparations _____

Quality Assurance

_____ 68. A built-in positive control to prove the device or test kit is working

_____ 69. The awareness and prevention of both the physical and procedural risks that may bring about an injury or legal action against the practice

_____ 70. A pattern of narrow and wide bars and spaces; each pattern is encoded with its own particular meaning

A. accuracy

B. Levy-Jennings chart

C. medical office risk management

____ 71. When both accuracy and precision are accomplished

____ 72. Liquid positive and negative controls that are tested the same way as the liquid patient specimen

____ 73. Ability to produce the same test result each time a test is performed (results are seen clustered together on a target)

____ 74. The average test result of a series of controls

____ 75. A statistical term describing the amount of variation from the mean in a dataset

____ 76. When controls consistently fall within the two standard deviations of the mean (results are seen within the center of a target)

____ 77. Used to plot the daily results of the control samples

D. bar codes

E. reliability

F. standard deviation

G. precision

H. internal control

I. external controls

J. mean

78. Compare the 10 areas of good laboratory practices for certificate of waiver laboratories (Figure 1-31 in the text) with the flow chart of the three phases of laboratory testing requiring quality assessment (Table 1-8 in the text) and draw lines between the good laboratory practices numbers, dividing them into the three phases of preanalytical, analytical, and postanalytical. Where should the lines be placed?

_____

_____

79. Quality assurance would oversee what area(s) of good laboratory practices? Quality control would take place during what area(s) of good laboratory practices?

_____

_____

80. What is the difference between qualitative tests and quantitative tests, and how does it affect quality control?

_____

_____

_____

81. Explain the relation of accuracy, precision, and reliability when plotting the results of standard controls.

_____

_____

_____

_____

82. Plot 4 weeks of daily glucose control results below on the four blank Levy-Jennings graphs. Mark the results for each day on the graph; in the blank provided, identify if the test system is experiencing a *trend*, a *shift*, a *random error*, or is *out of control*.

WEEK 1: day 1 = 103, day 2 = 100, day 3 = 98, day 4 = 112, day 5 = 105, day 6 = 99

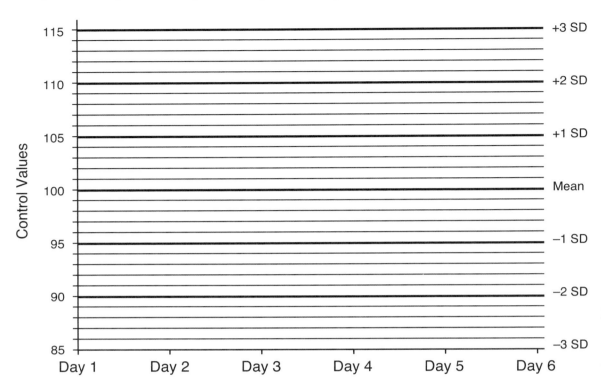

Week 1 glucose results: _____

WEEK 2: day 1 = 94, day 2 = 92, day 3 = 93, day 4 = 108, day 5 = 109, day 6 = 107

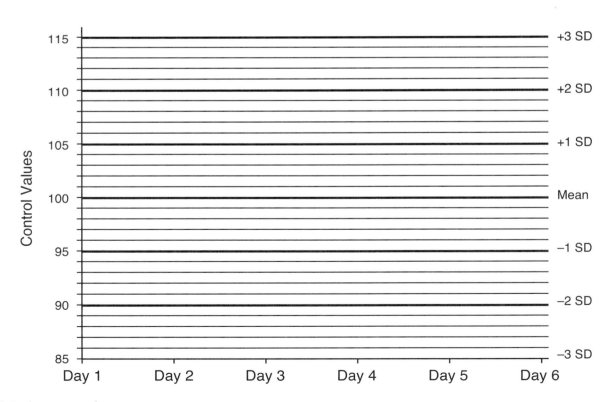

Week 2 glucose results: _____

Skill Procedure: Preparing Microscope for Examination

Person evaluated _____   Date _____

Evaluated by _____   Score/grade _____

Outcome goal	To bring a stained slide into focus from low power to high dry power and then focus on oil immersion
Conditions	Given a microscope, lens paper, a stained slide, immersion oil, and soft, lint-free tissue
Standards	Time = 15 minutes
	Accuracy = each step on check sheet is completed and an image is focused on oil immersion for evaluator check-off before cleanup

Evaluation Rubric Codes:

S = Satisfactory, meets standard   **U** = Unsatisfactory, fails to meet standard

Total possible points = _____   Points earned = _____

NOTE: Steps marked with an * are critical to achieve required competency.

Preparation	Scores	
	S	**U**
1. Carry microscope with two hands, uncover, and adjust for cleaning		
- One hand under base and the other grasping the arm of the scope		
2. Turn coarse focus until stage and objectives are farthest apart		
3. Clean ocular and all objective lenses with lens paper (clean oil lens last)		
4. Turn nosepiece to low power (the shortest tube)		
- Do not push on objective tubes; use the nosepiece to turn		
5. Adjust light settings		
- Bring condenser all the way up for stained specimen		
- Open iris diaphragm all the way with lever		
6. Position a stained slide over light source		
- Place slide with stained side up into mechanical holder clamp		
- By using mechanical control, move slide until stained area is above the light		
7. Adjust ocular lens to line up with eyes		

Procedure	Scores	
	S	**U**
Low Power Focus		
8. While looking through oculars, turn coarse adjustment until color starts to appear, then turn slowly to bring image into coarse focus		
- Note: always start with low power objective to avoid breaking slide		
- Tip: move the slide back and forth slightly with mechanical controls to pick up movement		
9. Move hand to fine focus adjustment, then turn one way and then the other until image becomes clear		
- Make sure both eyes are seeing a clear image; if not, adjust the oculars by turning their individual focus controls		
10. Move the slide to a place of interest in the center of the visual field, then turn the nosepiece to high power		
High Power Focus		
11. Refocus image by turning the fine adjustment one way and then the other until color is seen; then slowly bring in a clear image		
Note: do not use coarse adjustment because it will make too drastic a change and possibly break the slide. If the fine adjustment cannot focus, go back to low power and start again with the coarse and fine focus adjustments.		
- Move slide so that something interesting is in the middle		

Oil Immersion Preparation and Focus		
12. Turn the nosepiece halfway between high power and the oil immersion objective		
13. Place a drop of oil directly on the slide where the condenser light is shining		
14. Carefully turn the nosepiece until the oil immersion lens dips into the oil and snaps into place		
*15. While looking into the oculars, move the small fine focus adjustment back and forth until the image pops into view		
* When image is in view, obtain instructor verification. _____		
- Scan slide to see cells or organisms		
- Use one hand on the mechanical control to move slide and other hand on the fine focus to continuously make adjustments		

Follow-up	Scores	
	S	U
Cleanup and Microscope Maintenance		
16. Turn off the light and turn the nosepiece back to the low power objective		
- Turn coarse focus knob to maximize the distance between lens and stage		
- Remove slide and clean the stage with soft, lint-free tissue		
- Clean oil off the slide with the tissue or xylene		
17. With lens paper, clean off the ocular lenses and objective lenses, with the oil immersion lens always being the last to be cleaned		
*18. Cover the microscope with a dustproof cover and store in a clean, protected area.		
Total Points Per Column		

* The instructor or supervisor will verify a successfully focused result. This step is critical to achieve required competency.

Analytical Testing

Qualitative Test: _____

Person evaluated _____ Date _____

Evaluated by _____ Score/grade _____

Outcome goal	
Conditions	Supplies required:
Standards	**Required time** = _____ **minutes** **Performance time** = _____ **Total possible points** = _____ Points earned = _____
Evaluation Rubric Codes:	
S = Satisfactory, meets standard	**U** = Unsatisfactory, fails to meet standard
NOTE: Steps marked with an **✱** are critical to achieve required competency.	

Preparation: Preanalytical Phase	Scores	
	S	**U**
A. Test information		
- Kit method		
- Manufacturer		
- Proper storage (temp, light, etc.)		
- Lot number of kit _____		
- Expiration date _____		
- Package insert and/or test flow chart available: _____ yes _____ no		
B. Personal protective equipment		
C. Specimen Information		

Procedure: Analytical Phase	Scores	
	S	**U**
D. Performed/observed qualitative quality control		
- External liquid controls: Positive _____ Negative _____		
- Internal control:		

E. Performed patient test
1.
2.
3.
4.
POSITIVE seen as: NEGATIVE seen as: INVALID seen as:

* Accurate Results _____   Instructor Confirmation _____

Follow-up/Postanalytical Phase	Scores	
	S	U
* F. Proper documentation		
1. On control/patient log _____ yes _____ no		
2. Documentation on patient chart – See below		
3. Identified "critical values" and took appropriate steps to notify physician **EXPECTED VALUES FOR ANALYTE:**		
G. Proper disposal and disinfection		
1. Disposed all sharps into biohazard sharps containers		
2. Disposed all other regulated medical waste into biohazard bags		
3. Disinfected test area and instruments according to OSHA guidelines		
4. Sanitized hands after removing gloves		
Total Points Per Column		

Documentation on Patient Chart: Patient Name: _____

Patient Chart Entry: (Don't forget to include when, what, why, any additional information, and the signature of the person charting.)

_____

_____

Analytical Testing

Quantitative Test: _____

Person evaluated _____   Date _____

Evaluated by _____   Score/grade _____

Outcome goal	
Conditions	
Standards	**Required time** = _____ **minutes** **Performance time** = _____ **Total possible points** = _____ Points earned= _____
Evaluation Rubric Codes: **S** = Satisfactory, meets standard	**U** = Unsatisfactory, fails to meet standard
NOTE: Steps marked with an * are critical to achieve required competency.	

Preparation: Preanalytical Phase	Scores	
	S	**U**
A. Test information		
- Kit or instrument method _____		
- Manufacturer _____		
- Proper storage (temp, light, etc.) _____		
- Lot number of kit or supplies _____		
- Expiration date _____		
- Package insert and/or test flow chart available: _____ yes _____ no		
B. Specimen information		
- Type of specimen and its preparation (i.e. fasting, first morning, etc.) _____		
- Specimen container or testing device _____		
- Amount of specimen: _____		
C. Personal protective equipment		
D. Assembled all the above, sanitized hands, and applied PPE		
Procedure: Analytical Phase	**Scores**	
	S	**U**
E. Performed/observed quality control for A. or B. below		
Quantitative testing controls		
- Calibration check _____		
- Control levels: Normal _____ High _____ Low _____		
F. Performed patient test		
Followed proper steps (see test flow chart and list): _____		
1.		
2.		

3.	
4.	
5.	
6.	
7.	
8.	
9.	
10.	

* Accurate Results _____   Instructor Confirmation _____

Follow-Up/Postanalytical Phase	Scores	
	S	U
* G. Proper documentation		
1. On control log _____ yes _____ no		
2. On patient log _____ yes _____ no		
3. Documentation on patient chart – See below		
4. Identified "critical values" and took appropriate steps to notify physician EXPECTED VALUES FOR ANALYTE:		
H. Proper disposal and disinfection		
1. Dispose all sharps into biohazard sharp containers		
2. Dispose all other regulated medical waste into biohazard bags		
3. Disinfect test area and instruments according to OSHA guidelines		
4. Sanitize hands after removing gloves		
Total Points Per Column		

Documentation on Patient Chart: Patient Name: _____

Patient Chart Entry: (Don't forget to include when, what, why, any additional information, and the signature of the person charting.)

_____

_____

Urinalysis

VOCABULARY REVIEW

Match the following anatomic terms with their functions.

_____ 1. The functional unit of the kidney

_____ 2. Part of the nephron that contains the glomerulus and glomerular capsule

_____ 3. Structure in the renal corpuscle made up of tangled blood capillaries in which the hydrostatic pressure in the capillaries pushes substances through the capillary pores

_____ 4. Cup-shaped structure surrounding the glomerulus that collects the glomerular filtrate

_____ 5. Urethral opening through which urine is expelled

_____ 6. Slender, muscular tubes 10 to 12 inches long that carry the urine formed in the kidneys to the urinary bladder

_____ 7. Hollow muscular organ that holds urine until it is expelled

_____ 8. Tube that carries urine outside the body

_____ 9. Located behind the peritoneal cavity

_____ 10. Parts of the nephron composed of proximal convoluted tubules, the nephron loop (loop of Henle), and distal convoluted tubules

A. urethral meatus

B. glomerulus

C. glomerular capsule

D. urinary bladder

E. renal tubules

F. nephron

G. renal corpuscle

H. ureters

I. retroperitoneal

J. urethra

Match the following urinalysis terms with their definitions.

_____ 11. electrolyte

_____ 12. renal threshold level

_____ 13. oliguria

_____ 14. bilirubin

_____ 15. anuria

_____ 16. dysuria

_____ 17. nocturia

_____ 18. diuresis

_____ 19. porphyrin

_____ 20. glycosuria

_____ 21. reducing substances

_____ 22. ketonuria

A. Caused by treatment or diagnostic procedures

B. Substance that easily loses electrons

C. Intact red blood cells in the urine

D. Protein found in the urine of patients with multiple myeloma

E. Painful urination

F. Red cells breaking open and releasing hemoglobin

G. Expelling of urine, also referred to as voiding and urination

H. In urinalysis, the weight of urine compared with the weight of an equal volume of water; measures the amount of dissolved substances in urine

I. No urine flow

J. Sugars (especially glucose) in the urine

K. To break open

L. Decreased urine volume

_____ 23. hematuria

_____ 24. lyse

_____ 25. hemolysis

_____ 26. proteinuria

_____ 27. pyuria

_____ 28. iatrogenic

_____ 29. lipiduria

_____ 30. casts

_____ 31. micturition

_____ 32. pH

_____ 33. specific gravity

_____ 34. Bence Jones protein

M. Ketones in the urine

N. Excessive urination at night

O. Intermediate substance in the formation of heme (part of hemoglobin)

P. An element or compound that forms ions when dissolved and is able to conduct electricity

Q. Proteins in the urine

R. Lipids in the urine

S. Increase in the volume of urine output

T. Waste product from the breakdown of hemoglobin

U. White blood cells in the urine

V. Elements excreted in the urine in the shape of the renal tubules and ducts

W. Blood reabsorption limit of a substance and the point at which the substance is then excreted in the urine

X. Scale that measures the level of acidity or alkalinity of a solution

FUNDAMENTAL CONCEPTS

Anatomy of the Urinary System

35. Label the structures of the urinary system.

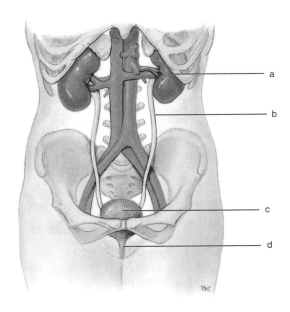

36. Label the structures of the kidney.

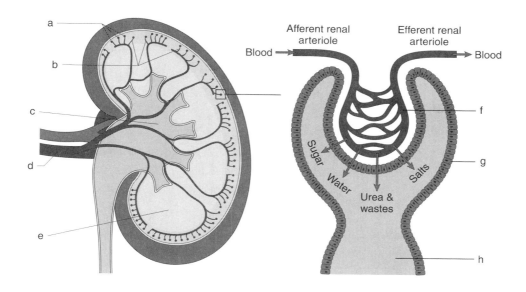

37. List three functions of the urinary system.

    1. _____

    2. _____

    3. _____

38. Describe the location of the kidneys in the body.

    _____

    _____

39. List the functions of the nephron.

    _____

    _____

40. Name the two structural components of the nephron.

    _____

    _____

41. List and describe the components of the renal corpuscle.

    _____

    _____

42. Describe the three steps of urine formation.

_____

_____

_____

43. Describe the term renal threshold.

_____

_____

44. Discuss the importance of a urinalysis.

_____

_____

45. Name the three parts of a urinalysis.

_____

_____

Urine Specimen Collection

46. Discuss the advantages of the first morning specimen.

_____

_____

_____

_____

47. Give three general requirements for all types of urine collection methods.

_____

_____

48. Discuss the proper handling and discarding of urine specimens.

_____

_____

49. When educating a female patient on the steps involved in preparing for midstream clean catch urine, why must the patient understand the importance of wiping from front to back?

_____

_____

_____

CLIA WAIVED URINALYSIS TESTS

Physical Urinalysis

50. Name the tests that are part of the physical urinalysis.

_____

_____

51. List the terms used to describe the appearance of urine.

_____

_____

52. Give the range of normal color for urine.

_____

_____

53. In what condition can urine have a sweet or fruity odor?

_____

_____

54. Discuss three abnormal urine colors, including the causes.

_____

_____

55. Describe the relevance of the specific gravity test in the urinalysis.

_____

_____

Chemical Urinalysis

56. Discuss the difference between qualitative, quantitative, and semiquantitative testing.

_____

_____

57. Label the urinalysis chemistry supplies (see Figure 2-10 in textbook).

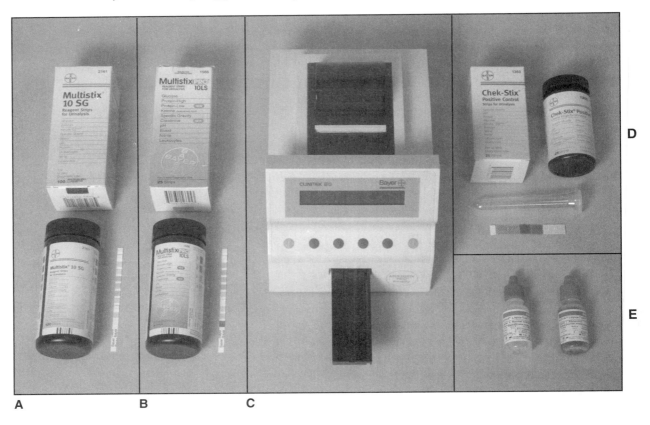

A   B   C

58. Name the 10 urinalysis chemistry tests that are most frequently performed.

1. _____   6. _____

2. _____   7. _____

3. _____   8. _____

4. _____   9. _____

5. _____   10. _____

59. Discuss the reasons for the new method that tests for microalbumin.

_____

_____

_____

60. List three conditions that may cause blood to be found in urine.

_____

_____

_____

61. Explain why a first morning urine sample is recommended when testing for nitrites.

_____

_____

62. If the nitrite test is negative, could bacteria be present in the urine?

_____

_____

63. Name a confirmatory test that can be performed when a urine sample is positive for the bilirubin test.

_____

_____

64. Describe the Clinitek instrument, including its advantages and disadvantages.

_____

_____

65. List three of the urinalysis chemistry reagent strip guidelines.

_____

_____

66. Describe the quality control methods available for urinalysis chemistry testing.

_____

_____

67. What would be the probable cause for the following urinalysis physical and chemical results, and what might the physician do next? Circle the abnormal results.
- Dark yellow
- Cloudy
- Glucose-neg
- Ketones-neg
- Bilirubin-neg
- Specific gravity 1.025
- pH 7
- Blood 2+
- Urobilinogen 0.2
- Protein-mod
- Nitrite-pos
- Leukocyte-mod

_____

_____

_____

68. What would be the probable cause for the following urinalysis chemical results? Circle the abnormal results.
    - Glucose 2%
    - Ketones-mod
    - Bilirubin-neg
    - Specific gravity 1.025
    - pH 6
    - Blood-neg
    - Urobilinogen 0.2
    - Protein-trace
    - Nitrite-neg
    - Leukocyte-neg

    _____

    _____

69. An abnormal urinalysis chemical control was performed with Bayer reagent strips and tablets. The following results were obtained. Circle the analyte(s) that are **not** in control range for the following results.
    Glucose- neg
    Bilirubin–pos
    Ketones–pos
    Specific gravity 1.015
    Blood large
    pH 8.5
    Protein 100 mg/dL
    Urobilinogen 3 mg/dL
    Nitrate–pos
    Leukocytes–mod

Test	Expected Results with Bayer Reagent Strips and Tablets	
	Chek-Stix Positive Control	**Chek-Stix Negative Control**
Glucose	100-250 mg/dL	Negative
Bilirubin	Positive	Negative
Ketone	Positive	Negative
Specific gravity	1.000-1.015 (adjusted for pH)	1.010-1.025 (adjusted for pH)
Blood	Moderate, large	Negative
pH	≥ 8.0	6.0-7.0
Protein	Trace, 100 mg/dL (SI units: trace, 1.0 g/L)	Negative
Urobilinogen	≥ 2 mg/dL	0.2-1 mg/dL
Nitrite	Positive	Negative
Leukocytes	Trace, moderate	Negative
Microbumintest	Positive (by using 1:3 dilution of Chek-Stix Positive control solution)	Negative
Acetest	Positive	Negative
Clinitest	250-750 mg/dL	Negative
Ictotest	Positive	Negative

ADVANCED CONCEPTS: MICROSCOPIC EXAMINATION URINALYSIS

70. In the standardized urinalysis Kova System for preparation of the microscopic examination, define the terms sediment and supernatant and state which of these is used in the microscopic examination of urine.

_____

_____

71. Describe the advantages of Sternheimer-Malbin stain.

_____

_____

72. List conditions in which _Candida albicans_ (yeast) may be found in the urine.

_____

_____

73. Name the four factors that can lead to cast formation.

_____

_____

74. Name the crystals that resemble envelopes (with an X appearance).

_____

_____

75. What part of the microscopic urinalysis can be performed by a medical assistant?

_____

_____

76. In the procedure for calculating a microscopic urinalysis:

a. What substances are observed on low power in a microscopic urinalysis?

_____

b. How many fields are observed on high power?

_____

c. Explain how substances are averaged and reported.

_____

77. Match the pictures of urine cells, casts, and crystals with their microscopic drawings. NOTE: Refer to photos and drawings on pp. 69-75 in your textbook, Figures 2-13 through 2-32.

Cells:

Word list: RBCs on high power, squamous epithelial cells on high power, transitional epithelial cells on high power, WBCs on high power

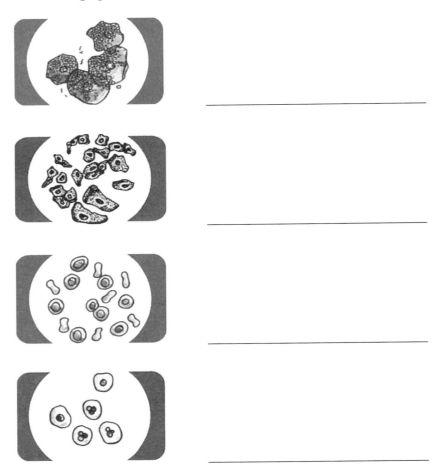

_____

_____

_____

_____

Casts:

Word list: granular casts, hyaline casts, RBC casts, WBC casts

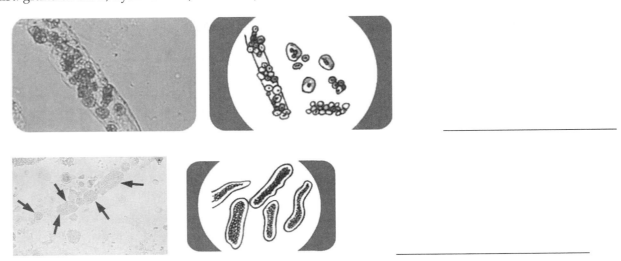

_____

_____

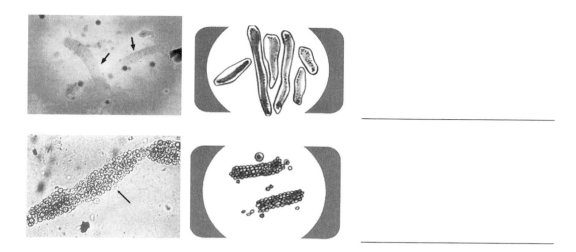

_____

_____

Crystals and others:

Word list: calcium oxalate crystals, _Trichomonas vaginalis_, triple phosphate crystals, yeast

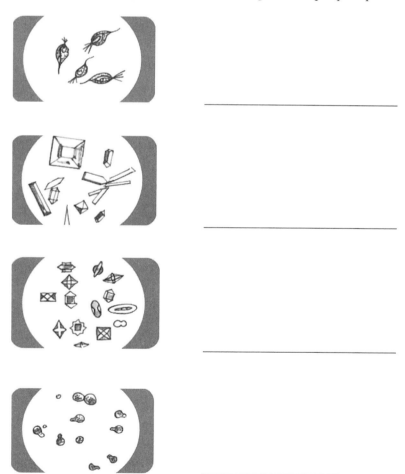

_____

_____

_____

_____

Skill Procedure: Female Instructions for Midstream Clean Catch Collection

Person evaluated _____ Date _____

Evaluated by _____

Outcome goal	Instruct a female patient regarding the correct procedure for midstream clean catch specimen
Conditions	Given the following:
	- Sterile urine collection container and label
	- Antiseptic towelettes
Standards	Required time = 15 minutes
	Performance time = _____

Evaluation Rubric Codes:
S = Satisfactory, meets standard   **U** = Unsatisfactory, fails to meet standard

Total possible points = _____   Points earned = _____

NOTE: Steps marked with an * are critical to achieve required competency.

Preparation	Scores	
	S	U
1. Washed hands and gathered the appropriate equipment		
2. Greeted and identified the patient		

Procedure	Scores	
	S	U
3. Instructed patient to sanitize her hands and remove underwear		
4. Instructed patient to spread apart the labia to expose the urinary opening		
- Patient told to keep this area spread apart with the nondominant hand during the entire cleaning procedure		
5. Instructed patient to take one antiseptic towelette and clean one side of the urinary opening from front to back, stressing the importance of the direction		
- Patient told that cleaning in this direction will prevent anal organisms from being spread to the urinary opening		
6. Instructed patient to take another antiseptic towelette and clean other side of the urinary opening from front to back, stressing the importance of the direction		
7. Instructed patient using a third antiseptic towelette to wipe from front to back directly across the urinary opening, stressing the importance of the direction		
8. Instructed patient to continue to keep labia spread apart and to urinate a small amount (one third) into the toilet, being careful not to touch the inside of the sterile container		
- Patient told that the reason for a small amount urinated in the toilet is to flush away microorganisms that may be around the urinary opening		
9. Instructed patient to collect the second part of the urine sample into the sterile container		
- Student was able to state that this would collect the midstream portion of the urine specimen		
10. Instructed patient to urinate the last portion of the urine into the toilet		
11. Instructed patient to dry the area with a tissue		
12. Instructed the patient on the correct procedure after the specimen has been collected		
- Instructed the patient to carefully cap the specimen - Instructed patient to place specimen in a certain area after collected in an office setting or to refrigerate if collected at home		

Follow-up	Scores	
	S	U
13. After receiving the specimen from the patient, the sample was labeled correctly and the requisition was completed if required		
14. Washed hands		
*15. Procedure was charted correctly		
- Charted that female patient was given instructions for midstream clean catch urine collection - Receiving of specimen from patient was charted		
Total Points Per Column		

Patient Chart Entry: (Don't forget to include when, what, how, why, any additional information, and the signature of the person charting.)

_____

_____

_____

Skill Procedure: Male Instructions for Midstream Clean Catch Collection

Person evaluated _____   Date _____

Evaluated by _____

Outcome goal	Instruct a male patient in the correct procedure for midstream clean catch specimen
Conditions	Given:
	- Sterile urine collection container and label
	- Antiseptic towelettes
Standards	Required time = 15 minutes
	Performance time = _____
Evaluation Rubric Codes:	
S = Satisfactory, meets standard **U** = Unsatisfactory, fails to meet standard	
Total possible points = _____ Points earned = _____	
NOTE: Steps marked with an **✱** are critical to achieve required competency.	

Preparation	Scores	
	S	U
1. Washed hands and gathered the appropriate equipment		
2. Greeted and identified the patient		

Procedure	Scores	
	S	U
3. Instructed patient to sanitize his hands and remove underwear		
4. If patient is uncircumcised, instructed the patient to retract the foreskin and hold it back during the entire procedure		
5. Instructed the patient to clean the area around the penis opening by starting at the tip of the penis and cleaning downward, using a separate antiseptic towelette for each side		
6. Instructed patient to use a third antiseptic towelette to clean across the opening		
✱7. Instructed patient to urinate a small amount (one third) into the toilet, being careful not to touch the inside of the sterile container		
- Patient told that the reason for a small amount urinated in the toilet is to flush away microorganisms that may be around the urinary opening		
8. Instructed patient to collect the second part of the urine sample into the sterile container		
- Student was able to state that this would collect the midstream portion of the urine specimen		
9. Instructed patient to urinate the last portion of the urine into the toilet		
10. Instructed patient to dry the area with a tissue if needed		

Follow-up	Scores	
	S	U
11. Instructed the patient on the correct procedure after the specimen has been collected		
- Instructed the patient to carefully cap the specimen - Instructed patient to place specimen in a certain area after collected in an office setting or to refrigerate if collected at home		

12. After receiving the specimen from the patient, the sample was labeled correctly and the requisition was completed if required		
13. Washed hands		
14. Procedure was charted correctly		
- Charted that male patient was given instructions for midstream clean catch urine collection		
- Receiving of specimen from patient was charted		
Total Points Per Column		

Patient Chart Entry: (Don't forget to include when, what, how, why, any additional information, and the signature of the person charting.)

_____

_____

_____

Skill Procedure: 24-Hour Urine Collection Instructions

Person evaluated _____   Date _____

Evaluated by _____

Outcome goal	To educate the patient on the correct instructions for collection of a 24-hour urine specimen
Conditions	Given: - Large urine container - Instructions sheet - Requisition
Standards	Required time = 15 minutes Performance time = _____
Evaluation Rubric Codes: **S** = Satisfactory, meets standard **U** = Unsatisfactory, fails to meet standard Total possible points = _____ Points earned = _____	
NOTE: Steps marked with an ✶ are critical to achieve required competency.	

Preparation	Scores	
	S	U
1. Washed hands and gathered the appropriate equipment		
2. Greeted and identified the patient		

Procedure	Scores	
	S	U
3. Instructed patient when arising on the first day of the 24-hour collection procedure to empty bladder into the toilet		
- Instructed patient to record this time		
4. Instructed the patient that all urine for 24 hours after that first voided specimen must be voided directly into the collection container		
- Informed the patient to be sure to screw the lid on tightly each time and keep the container refrigerated		
- Informed the patient that if at any time during the procedure some urine is not collected, the test will need to start again. Gave examples of this.		
5. Instructed the patient that on the second morning of the 24-hour period the patient must arise at the same time as the first day and urinate directly into the container, keeping this sample		
- Patient was instructed that the first morning specimen on the second day of the 24-hour period is the last sample collected and is the completion of the collection procedure		
6. Instructed the patient that on the day the procedure is completed the container must be returned to the physician's office or to the laboratory		

Follow-up	Scores	
	S	U
7. After the patient completed the procedure and returned the container, the patient was asked if any problems occurred during the collection procedure		
8. Completed a laboratory requisition form for test ordered		

9. Prepared the specimen to be transported to the laboratory that will perform the testing		
10. Charted the instructions and equipment supplied to the patient		
- When patient returned with specimen, charted that the specimen was sent to the laboratory, documenting all necessary information concerning the specimen		
Total Points Per Column		

Patient Chart Entry: (Don't forget to include when, what, how, why, any additional information, and the signature of the person charting.)

_____

_____

_____

Analytical Test: Refractometer Method for Determining Specific Gravity

Person evaluated _____   Date _____

Evaluated by _____

Outcome goal	Perform the refractometer method for specific gravity on an unknown sample according to stated task, conditions, and standards
Conditions	Given: - Refractometer instrument - Disposable pipette - Lens paper or soft wipes
Standards	Required time = 10 minutes Performance time = _____

Evaluation Rubric Codes:
S = Satisfactory, meets standard   **U** = Unsatisfactory, fails to meet standard

Total possible points = _____   Points earned = _____

NOTE: Steps marked with an **✱** are critical to achieve required competency.

Preparation: Preanalytical Phase	Scores	
	S	U
A. Test information		
- Kit or instrument method **refractometer method**		
B. Specimen information		
- Any urine specimen collected in clean container		
- Amount **one to two drops**		
C. Personal protective equipment **gloves and biohazard container**		

Procedure: Analytical Phase	Scores	
	S	U
D. Perform/observe quality control		
- Quantitative testing controls **use distilled water**		
- Control results **distilled water must equal 1.000**		
E. Performed patient test	S	U
1. Filled a small amount of urine in a disposable pipette by holding the pipette in a vertical position and placing a drop of urine on the prism; used the method required by the instrument being used to fill the well		
2. Pointed the refractometer toward a light source and rotated the eyepiece to bring the scale into clear view		
3. Correctly determined results by reading the specific gravity scale at the borderline between the dark and light areas		
✱Accurate Results _____ **Instructor Confirmation** _____		

Follow-up/Postanalytical Phase	Scores	
	S	U
✱F. Proper documentation _____		
1. On control log _____ yes _____ no		
2. On patient log _____ yes _____ no		
3. Documentation on patient chart; see below		

4. Identified critical values and took appropriate steps to notify physician Expected values for analyte: S/P = 1.005-1.025		
G. Proper disposal and disinfection		
1. Disposed all sharps into biohazard sharps containers		
2. Disposed all other regulated medical waste into biohazard bags		
3. Disinfected test area and instruments according to OSHA guidelines		
4. Sanitized hands after removing gloves		
Total Points Per Column		

Patient name: _____

Patient Chart Entry: (Don't forget to include when, what, how, why, any additional information, and the signature of the person charting.)

_____

_____

_____

Analytical Test: Clinitest

Person evaluated _____   Date _____

Evaluated by _____

Outcome goal	Perform a Clinitest test on an unknown sample
Conditions	Given: - Clinitest bottle of tablets - Clinitest tube - Tube of water with pipette - Urine sample with pipette - Clinitest reference chart
Standards	Required time = 15 minutes Performance time = _____

Evaluation Rubric Codes:

S = Satisfactory, meets standard   **U** = Unsatisfactory, fails to meet standard

Total possible points = _____   Points earned = _____

NOTE: Steps marked with an ✽ are critical to achieve required competency

Preparation: Preanalytical Phase	Scores	
	S	U
A. Test information		
- Kit or instrument method **Clinitest**		
- Manufacturer **Bayer Corporation**		
- Proper storage (temperature, light, etc.) **room temperature with the lid tightly sealed; protect tablets from light, heat, and moisture**		
- Lot number of kit _____		
- Expiration date _____		
- Package insert available _____ yes _____ no		
B. Specimen information		
- Labeled urine specimen in clean container		
- Amount **2 or 5 drops (according to directions)**		
C. Personal protective equipment **gloves, sharps, and biohazard**		

Procedure: Analytical Phase	Scores	
	S	U
D. Performed/observed quality control		
1. Semiquantitative testing controls		
- Control levels: Normal _____ Abnormal _____		
E. Performed patient test	S	U
1. Added 5 drops of urine to 10 drops of water in a Clinitest tube		
2. Tapped the Clinitest tablet into the tube, which was placed in a rack because the boiling reaction that occurs is very hot		
3. During the boiling reaction, the tube was observed for any color change		
- The boiling reaction should be observed for the "pass through effect," which results with color change occurring during the reaction and appears negative when the reaction is completed and results are determined		

	Scores	
	S	U
4. Shook the tube 15 seconds after the boiling had stopped to mix the contents		
5. Compared color of the reaction with the Clinitest chart for the 5-drop method and recorded the results		

*Accurate Results _____ Instructor Confirmation _____

Follow-up: Postanalytical Phase	Scores	
	S	U
*F. Proper documentation_____		
1. On control log _____ yes _____ no		
2. On patient log _____ yes _____ no		
3. Documentation on patient chart (see below)		
4. Identified critical values and took appropriate steps to notify physician Expected values for analyte **negative**		
G. Proper disposal and disinfection		
1. Disposed all other regulated medical waste into biohazard bags		
2. Disinfected test area and instruments according to OSHA guidelines		
3. Sanitized hands after removing gloves		
Total Points Per Column		

Patient name: _____

Patient Chart Entry: (Don't forget to include when, how, what, why, any additional information, and the signature of the person charting.)

_____

_____

_____

Skill Procedure: Urinalysis Microscopic Examination

Person evaluated _____   Date _____

Evaluated by _____

Outcome goal:	To prepare a microscopic urinalysis slide, focus the slide on the microscope, and state the elements that can be found under low and high power
Conditions	Given: - Gloves - Urine specimen - Kova equipment: cap, pipette - Sternheimer-Malbin stain - Test tube - Centrifuge - Microscope
Standards	Required time = 10 minutes Performance time = _____
Evaluation Rubric Codes: S = Satisfactory, meets standard U = Unsatisfactory, fails to meet standard Total possible points = _____ Points earned = _____	
NOTE: Steps marked with an * are critical to achieve required competency.	

Preparation	Scores	
	S	U
1. Washed hands, applied gloves, and gathered the appropriate equipment		
*2. Mixed the correctly identified room temperature urine specimen		
*3. Poured the urine sample to the "12" mark in a urine centrifuge tube and capped the tube		

Procedure	Scores	
	S	U
*4. Centrifuged the tube for 5 minutes at 1500 rpm		
- Stated the definition of sediment and supernatant		
*5. Carefully removed the spun tube from the centrifuge and removed the cap		
*6. Carefully placed the Kova pipette into the bottom of the tube		
- Hooked the clip on the top of the pipette over the outside of the tube		
*7. Placed index finger on tip of the pipette and decanted off the supernatant by inverting the tube		
- Stated the approximate amount of sediment that remained in the tube		
8. Removed the pipette from the tube, added a drop of stain, and reinserted the pipette, squeezing gently to mix the urine sediment and stain		
- Stated the purpose of using the stain		
*9. Correctly transferred a drop of the urine sediment to a well in a Kova slide		
- Did not overfill or underfill the well		
*10. Allowed the Kova slide to sit for 1 minute		
- Stated why the slide should sit		

	S	U
11. Stated who is qualified to perform a urine microscopic examination		
12. Demonstrated the ability to focus a slide on the microscope		
- Focused first with low power with the course adjustment		
- Was able to fine focus with the fine adjustment knob		
*13. Stated what elements are observed under low power		
*14. Stated what elements are observed under high power		
*Accurate Results _____ Instructor Confirmation _____		

Follow-up/Postanalytical	Scores	
	S	U
15. Demonstrated the proper procedure for cleaning, carrying, and storing the microscope		
16. Correctly discarded the equipment in the appropriate containers		
- Discarded the urine specimen in the appropriate manner		
17. Removed and discarded gloves in the appropriate biohazard containers		
18. Sanitized hands		
19. Demonstrated an understanding of the process for calculating a urinalysis microscopic examination		
Total Points Per Column		

Patient Chart Entry: (Don't forget to include when, what, how, why, any additional information, and the signature of the person charting.)

_____

_____

_____

Analytical Test: Physical and Chemical Urinalysis

Person evaluated _____   Date _____

Evaluated by _____

Outcome goal	Perform a physical and chemical test on an unknown sample according to stated conditions and standards
Conditions	Given: - Reagent strips - Timing device - Reference chart - Requisition
Standards	Required time: 10 minutes Performance time _____

Evaluation Rubric Codes:
S = Satisfactory, meets standard   **U** = Unsatisfactory, fails to meet standard

Total possible points = _____   Points earned = _____

Preparation: Preanalytical Phase	Scores	
	S	U
A. Test information		
- Kit or instrument method **Multistix 10 SG**		
- Manufacturer **Bayer Corporation**		
- Proper storage (temperature, light, etc.) **room temperature, no direct sunlight**		
- Expiration date _____		
- Lot number _____		
- Package insert or test flow chart ____ yes ____ no		
B. Proper specimen		
- Special patient preparation (e.g., fasting, special diet, first morning specimen) **no special preparation**		
- Appropriate container **clean container without preservatives**		
- Amount of specimen **25 to 50 ml well-mixed urine**		
C. Personal protective equipment **gloves, gown, and biohazard container**		

Procedure: Analytical Phase	Scores	
	S	U
*D. Performed/observed quality control methods		
1. Semiquantitative liquid controls		
- Control levels: Normal _____ Abnormal _____		
*E. Performed patient test	S	U
1. Hands were sanitized and equipment assembled		
2. Urine was poured into a clear container or centrifuge tube		
3. The color of the urine was determined		
4. The clarity of the urine was determined		
5. Strip was removed from the bottle and the bottle was immediately closed. The pads on the strip were not touched and the strip was held parallel to the chart.		
6. The pads were completely covered with urine. The pads were not immersed too long, which could cause the reagents to dissolve and leach out into the urine.		

7. After removing the strip from the urine, the strip was tapped against the side of the tube to remove excess urine		
8. The color of each strip pad was read at a particular time and compared to the reference chart		

*Accurate Results (see attached forms)   Instructor Confirmation _____

	Scores	
Follow-up: Postanalytical Phase	**S**	**U**

*F. Proper documentation _____		
1. On control log _____ yes _____ no		
2. On patient log _____ yes _____ no		
3. Documentation on patient chart forms on next page		
4. Identified critical values and took appropriate steps to notify physician		

Analyte Expected Values

Glucose	**neg**
Bilirubin	**neg**
Ketone	**neg**
Specific gravity	**1.005-1.030**
Blood	**neg**
pH	**6.0-8.0**
Protein	**neg/trace**
Urobilirubin	**norm**
Nitrite	**neg**
Leukocytes	**neg**

G. Proper disposal and disinfection		
1. Disposed all sharps into biohazard sharps containers		
2. Disposed all other regulated medical waste into biohazard bags		
3. Disinfected test area and instruments according to OSHA guidelines		
4. Sanitized hands after removing gloves		
Total Points Per Column		

Forms for documentation on patient charts:

Patient:						Date/Time Spec. Collected:							
Doctor:			DOB:			Date/Time Spec. Completed:							
☐ VOID	TEST	REFERENCE	RESULT	TEST	REFERENCE	RESULT		TEST	REFERENCE	RESULT	TEST	REFERENCE	RESULT
	Color	Yellow		Blood	Neg			WBC	0 - 5 HPF		Bact.	0 - 5	
☐ CC	Char.	Clear		pH	5.0 - 8.0			RBC	0 - 3 HPF		Mucus	0	
☐ CATH	Glucose	Neg		Protein	Neg		MICRO	Epith.	D		Casts	0	
☐ TURBID	Bilirubin	Neg		Urobili	0.2 - 1.0 EU			Cryst.	0 - 3 HPF				
☐ HAZY	Ketone	Neg		Nitrite	Neg		OTHER:						
☐ CLEAR	Sp. Gr	1,000-1,030		Leuk	Neg								

Patient:						Date/Time Spec. Collected:							
Doctor:			DOB:			Date/Time Spec. Completed:							
☐ VOID	TEST	REFERENCE	RESULT	TEST	REFERENCE	RESULT		TEST	REFERENCE	RESULT	TEST	REFERENCE	RESULT
	Color	Yellow		Blood	Neg			WBC	0 - 5 HPF		Bact.	0 - 5	
☐ CC	Char.	Clear		pH	5.0 - 8.0			RBC	0 - 3 HPF		Mucus	0	
☐ CATH	Glucose	Neg		Protein	Neg		MICRO	Epith.	D		Casts	0	
☐ TURBID	Bilirubin	Neg		Urobili	0.2 - 1.0 EU			Cryst.	0 - 3 HPF				
☐ HAZY	Ketone	Neg		Nitrite	Neg		OTHER:						
☐ CLEAR	Sp. Gr	1,000-1,030		Leuk	Neg								

Patient:						Date/Time Spec. Collected:							
Doctor:			DOB:			Date/Time Spec. Completed:							
☐ VOID	TEST	REFERENCE	RESULT	TEST	REFERENCE	RESULT		TEST	REFERENCE	RESULT	TEST	REFERENCE	RESULT
	Color	Yellow		Blood	Neg			WBC	0 - 5 HPF		Bact.	0 - 5	
☐ CC	Char.	Clear		pH	5.0 - 8.0			RBC	0 - 3 HPF		Mucus	0	
☐ CATH	Glucose	Neg		Protein	Neg		MICRO	Epith.	D		Casts	0	
☐ TURBID	Bilirubin	Neg		Urobili	0.2 - 1.0 EU			Cryst.	0 - 3 HPF				
☐ HAZY	Ketone	Neg		Nitrite	Neg		OTHER:						
☐ CLEAR	Sp. Gr	1,000-1,030		Leuk	Neg								

Hematology

VOCABULARY REVIEW

Match the following hematology terms with their definitions.

A. anisocytosis

B. baso

C. differentiate

D. eosin

E. erythroblasts

F. formed elements

G. granulocytes

H. hematologists

I. hematopoiesis

J. hemocytoblast

K. macrophages

L. megakaryocyte

M. myeloblast

N. nongranulocytes

O. -phil

P. poikilocytosis

Q. polymorphonuclear

R. reticulocytes

S. thrombocytes

____ 1. A large nuclear cell in the bone marrow that fragments its cytoplasm to become platelets

____ 2. A stem cell that develops into the three kinds of granulocytes

____ 3. Abnormally shaped

____ 4. Acid

____ 5. Alkaline

____ 6. Also called rubriblasts, which become red blood cells

____ 7. Attraction

____ 8. Blood production

____ 9. Cells and cell fragments that can be viewed under the microscope

____ 10. Specialists who evaluate the cellular elements of blood microscopically and analytically

____ 11. Large, engulfing cells in the tissues that come from monocytes

____ 12. Lymphocyte and monocyte group

____ 13. Many-shaped nucleus; also called PMN or seg

____ 14. Neutrophils, basophils, and eosinophils group

____ 15. Newly released red blood cells in the blood that still contain some nuclear DNA

____ 16. Stem cell capable of becoming any of the blood cells

____ 17. To change and become something different

____ 18. Variances in red blood cell size

____ 19. Platelets

Match the following coagulation and pathological terms.

A. anemia	G. leukemia	M. rouleaux formation
B. embolus	H. leukocytosis	N. thrombosis
C. fibrinogen, prothrombin	I. leukopenia	O. vitamin K
D. hemolysis	J. polycythemia	P. differential count
E. hemostasis	K. red blood cell indices	Q. polychromia
F. hypoxemia	L. coagulation	

_____ 20. A critical element in the production of prothrombin

_____ 21. A traveling clot

_____ 22. Abnormal condition of increased red blood cells

_____ 23. Abnormal decrease in white blood cells

_____ 24. Abnormal increase in white blood cells

_____ 25. Abnormal condition of clotting

_____ 26. Condition in which the red blood cell or hemoglobin levels are below normal

_____ 27. Destruction of the red blood cells

_____ 28. Lack of oxygen in the blood

_____ 29. Like stacked chips

_____ 30. Mathematic ratios of the three red blood cell tests (hemoglobin, hematocrit, and red blood cell count)

_____ 31. The blood's ability to maintain the balance of initiating a clotting response to stop bleeding and at the same time prevent the blood from forming an unwanted stationary clot

_____ 32. Two plasma proteins involved in clotting

_____ 33. Percentage of the five different kinds of white blood cells

_____ 34. Cancer of the white blood cells

_____ 35. Increase in color (based on hemoglobin concentration)

_____ 36. Process of clotting

FUNDAMENTAL CONCEPTS

37. Blood collected from a _____ or a _____ may be used for routine hematologic procedures.

38. The anticoagulated Vacutainer tube containing _____ with a _____ top is used for most hematology tests.

39. Match the blood components below with their associated characteristic.

_____ basophil   A. Able to engulf foreign matter, especially bacteria

_____ erythrocyte   B. Increases in number during allergic reactions

_____ monocyte   C. Can differentiate into a T cell or B cell

_____ neutrophil   D. Enters the tissues to mediate the inflammatory response

_____ platelet   E. Gathers around the site of a damaged blood vessel and releases chemicals to stimulate clot formation

_____ lymphocyte   F. Carries oxygen from the lungs to the cells of the body

_____ eosinophil   G. Becomes a macrophage when it leaves the blood to clean up debris in the tissues

40. Label the missing elements of the following hematopoiesis chart (see Figure 4-3 in the text).

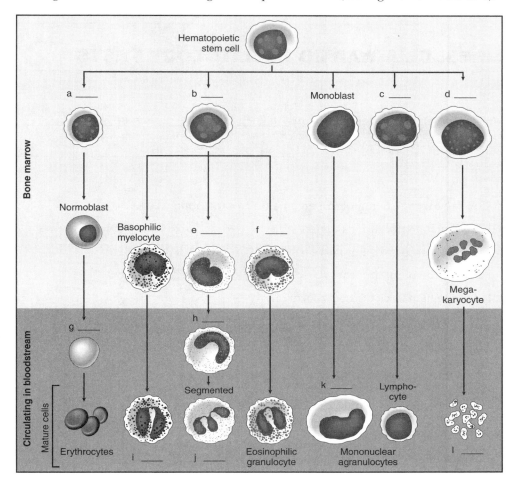

Preparation of a Blood Smear

41. A properly done blood smear will have a _____ edge at the thin end of the slide and a section containing well-distributed blood cells in the _____ of the slide.

42. Blood smears are observed under the _____ lens.

43. When identifying cells, what three characteristics should the technician observe? (Hint: Figure 4-22 displays the three general characteristics to observe in red cells.)

_____

_____

Hemostasis

44. Explain the involvement of each of the following as they pertain to hemostasis.

Blood vessels _____

Platelets _____

Clotting factors _____

Anticoagulants _____

45. What is the difference between a thrombus and an embolus? _____

_____

PROCEDURES: CLIA WAIVED HEMATOLOGY TESTS

Hemoglobin

46. The two main components of hemoglobin are _____ and _____.

47. What is the function of hemoglobin? _____

Hematocrit

48. Match the following average hematocrit percentages to each population.

   ____ Normal average hematocrit for women   a. 56%

   ____ Normal average hematocrit for a 6-year-old child   b. 42%

   ____ Normal average hematocrit for men   c. 38%

   ____ Normal average hematocrit for newborns   d. 47%

49. If a sample of capillary blood is used for the microhematocrit, the capillary tube must contain a(n) _____.

50. One condition in which a low hematocrit value might be found is _____.

51. True or false: Spun hematocrits should be performed in duplicate. _____

52. Label the layers of the spun hematocrit tube.

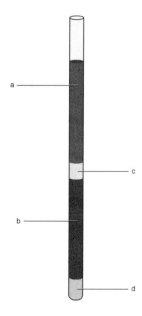

Erythrocyte Sedimentation Rate

53. What medical conditions would cause an increased erythrocyte sedimentation rate?

_____

_____

54. What technical interferences would cause an increased erythrocyte sedimentation rate?

_____

_____

Prothrombin Time

55. Describe the role of prothrombin in blood coagulation.

_____

_____

56. Explain the major use of the prothrombin time test. _____

_____

_____

57. Match the following tests with their reference ranges.

____ hemoglobin   a. 36% to 55%

____ hematocrit   b. 0 to 20 mm/hr

____ ProTime   c. 12 to 18 g/dL

____ ESR   d. 16 to 18 seconds or 2.0 to 2.5 INR

58. Label the Hemocue equipment and supplies (see Procedure 4-2 in textbook).

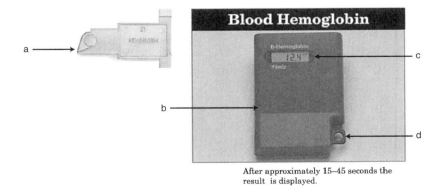

After approximately 15–45 seconds the result is displayed.

59. Label the HemataSTAT equipment and supplies (see Procedure 4-3 in textbook).

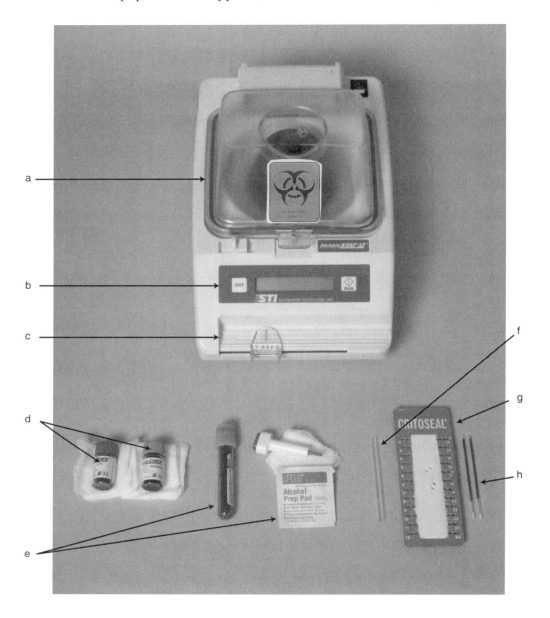

60. Label the SEDIPLAST ESR supplies (see Procedure 4-4 in textbook).

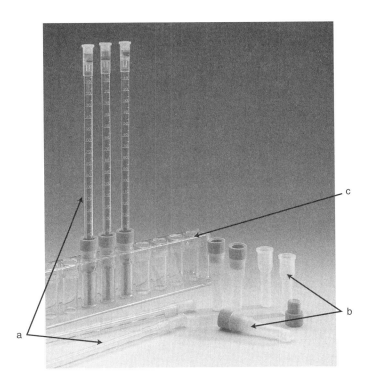

61. Label the ProTime equipment and supplies (see Procedure 4-5 in textbook).

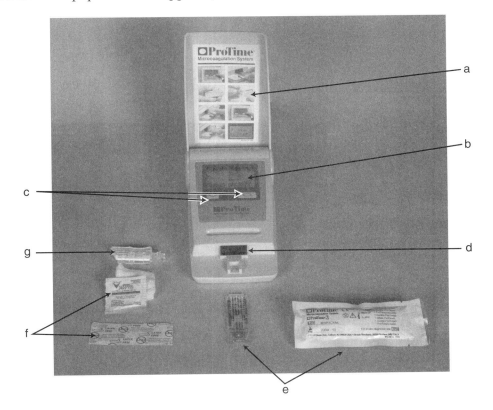

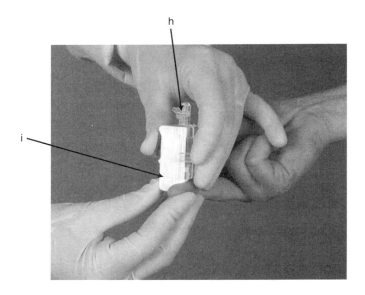

ADVANCED CONCEPTS: COMPLETE BLOOD COUNT

62. List the seven tests involved in the complete blood count.

_____

_____

_____

63. What changes in blood cell size are caused by deficiency of vitamin B_{12}? (Hint: Look under "Anemias" in text.)

_____

_____

64. List two conditions in which anisocytosis is found. (Hint: Also found under "Anemias.")

_____

_____

65. Match the red blood cell indexes to their reference ranges. (Hint: See Table 4-4 or 4-5 and note the units associated with each test.)

_____ MCV   a. 26 to 34 pg

_____ MCH   b. 31% to 37% or g/dL

_____ MCHC   c. 82 to 98 μm^3 or fL

66. Hypochromic, microcytic red blood cells have a (higher or lower) _____ MCV and (higher or lower) _____ MCHC.

67. Why does anemia and/or thrombocytopenia develop in patients with leukemia? (Hint: Consider where and how hematopoiesis occurs.)

_____

_____

68. Name one cause of eosinophilia. (Review granulocyte functions in Fundamental Concepts.)

_____

_____

69. Name one cause of neutrophilia. (Review granulocyte functions in Fundamental Concepts.)

_____

_____

70. Match the cell with its differential reference percentage according to Table 4-4.

_____ band   a. 3% to 9%

_____ lymphocyte   b. 50% to 65%

_____ neutrophil   c. 0% to 7%

_____ monocyte   d. 0% to 1%

_____ eosinophil   e. 25% to 40%

_____ basophil   f. 1% to 3%

Analytical Test: Hemocue Test for Blood Hemoglobin

Person evaluated _____   Date _____

Evaluated by _____

Outcome goal	Perform FDA-approved hemoglobin waived test following the most current OSHA safety guidelines and applying the correct quality control
Conditions	Given - Control cuvette - Microcuvette testing devices - Liquid controls: high and low - Alcohol, gauze, safety lancets, and bandage
Standards	Required time = 10 minutes Performance Time = _____ Total possible points = _____ Points earned = _____
Evaluation Rubric Codes: **S** = Satisfactory, meets standard **U** = Unsatisfactory, fails to meet standard	
NOTE: Steps marked with an ✱ are critical to achieve required competency.	

Preparation: Preanalytical Phase	Scores	
	S	**U**
A. Test information		
- Kit or instrument method **Hemocue hemoglobin**		
- Manufacturer **Hemocue**		
- Proper storage (temperature, light, etc.) **cuvettes stored at room temperature**		
- Lot number on cuvette container_____		
- Expiration date_____ **opened container is stable for 3 months**		
- Test flow chart _____ yes _____ no		
B. Specimen information		
- Type of specimen **capillary blood or EDTA tube blood**		
- Testing device **microcuvette test device**		
C. Personal protective equipment **gloves, gown, sharps, and biohazard**		
D. Assembled all the above, sanitized hands, and applied personal protective equipment		
Procedure: Analytical Phase	**Scores**	
	S	**U**
E. Performed/observed quality control		
1. Quantitative testing controls		
- Calibration check **used control cuvette for optics check**		
- Control levels: high _____ low _____		
F. Performed patient test	**S**	**U**
1. Followed proper steps (from test flow chart)		
2. Properly obtained sufficient drop of blood		
- Wiped away first drop and allowed new drop to form		
3. Filled cuvette completely in one continuous process; did not top off		

4. Wiped off excess blood on outside of cuvette immediately		
- Avoided pulling out blood by contacting tip of cuvette		
5. Visually inspected for air bubbles and loss of blood from cuvette		
6. Placed filled cuvette into the cuvette holder and pushed holder into the measuring position		
7. Result displayed after 30 to 60 seconds		

*Accurate Results _____   Instructor Confirmation _____

Follow-up/Postanalytical Phase	Scores	
	S	U
*G. Proper documentation		
1. On control log _____ yes _____ no		
2. On patient log _____ yes _____ no		
3. Documented on patient chart (see below)		
4. Identified critical values and took appropriate steps to notify physician		
- Hemoglobin expected values: Adult men = 13.0 to 18 g/dL Adult women = 11.0 to 16.0 g/dL Infants = 10.0 to 14.0 g/dL Children = increase to adult		
H. Proper disposal and disinfection		
1. Disposed all sharps into biohazard sharps containers		
2. Disposed all other regulated medical waste into biohazard bags		
3. Disinfected test area and instruments according to OSHA guidelines		
4. Sanitized hands after removing gloves		
Totals Counts per Column		

Patient name: _____

Patient Chart Entry: (Don't forget to include when, what, why, any additional information, and the signature of the person charting.)

_____

_____

_____

Analytical Test: Hematocrit (HemataSTAT Test)

Person evaluated _____   Date _____

Evaluated by _____

Outcome goal	Perform FDA-approved hematocrit waived test following the most current OSHA safety guidelines and applying the correct quality control
Conditions	Supplies required: - Plastic capillary pipettes with anticoagulant - Sealant clay (i.e., Critoseal) - Liquid controls: high and low - Gloves, gown, alcohol, gauze, and lancets
Standards	Required time = 15 minutes Performance time = _____ Total possible points = _____ Points earned = _____
Evaluation Rubric Codes: **S** = Satisfactory, meets standard **U** = Unsatisfactory, fails to meet standard	
NOTE: Steps marked with an **✱** are critical to achieve required competency.	

Preparation: Preanalytical Phase	Scores	
	S	U
A. Test information		
- Kit or instrument method **HemataSTAT-II**		
- Manufacturer **STI, Separation Technology, Inc.**		
- Proper storage (temperature, light, etc.) **room temperature**		
- Expiration date **(2 years, or 30 days after opened)**		
- Package insert or test flow chart available: _____ yes _____ no		
B. Specimen information		
- Type of specimen **capillary blood or venous blood in EDTA tube**		
- Specimen testing device **two capillary tubes filled at least halfway**		
C. Personal protective equipment **gloves, gown, face shield**		
D. Assembled all the above, sanitized hands, and applied personal protective equipment		

Procedure: Analytical Phase	Scores	
	S	U
E. Performed/observed quality control		
1. Quantitative testing controls		
- **HemataCHEK reference control**		
- Control levels: high _____ low _____ normal _____		
F. Perform patient test	S	U
1. Followed proper steps (from test flow chart)		
2. Collected whole blood into capillary tubes and sealed one end by pressing and turning in sealant, then tapped the sealed end		
3. Inserted the sealed end of capillary tube into the HemataSTAT rotor tube holder		
4. Closed centrifuge lid, locked latch, and pressed "RUN" to spin for 60 seconds		
5. Waited for beeps, then unlocked latch and opened lid		

6. Moved slider and sealed end of capillary tube to far left side of reader tray and rotated tube so entire "RED CELL/PLASMA" diagonal interface could be seen		
7. Pressed "ENT" to read tube		
8. Moved the slider black line to "SEALANT/RED CELL" interface and pressed "ENT"		
9. Moved the slider black line to "RED CELL/PLASMA" interface and pressed "ENT"		
10. Moved slider black line to "PLASMA/AIR" interface and pressed "ENT"		
11. Noted test result		
12. Repeated steps 4 to 9 with second tube:		
- Result must be within 2% agreement of first reading		
- Recorded the average of the two readings		

*Accurate Results _____   Instructor Confirmation _____

Follow-up/Postanalytical Phase	Scores	
	S	U
*G. Proper documentation		
1. On control log _____ yes _____ no		
2. On patient log _____ yes _____ no		
3. Documented on patient chart (see below)		
4. Identified critical values and took appropriate steps to notify physician		
- Hematocrit expected values: Adult men = 42% to 52% Adult women = 36% to 48% Infants = 32% to 38% Children = increase to adult		
H. Proper disposal and disinfection		
1. Disposed all sharps into biohazard sharps containers		
2. Disposed all other regulated medical waste into biohazard bags		
3. Disinfected test area and instruments according to OSHA guidelines		
4. Sanitized hands after removing gloves		
Totals Counts per Column		

Patient Name: _____

Patient Chart Entry: (Don't forget to include when, what, why, any additional information, and the signature of the person charting.)

_____

_____

Analytical Test: SEDIPLAST Erythrocyte Sedimentation Rate

Person evaluated _____   Date _____

Evaluated by _____

Outcome goal	Perform FDA-approved ESR waived test following the most current OSHA safety guidelines and applying the correct quality control
Conditions	Supplies needed: - Plastic Westergren pipette graduated from 0 to 200 mm - SEDIPLAST vials with citrate diluent - Westergren rack for holding the pipettes - Disposal transfer pipette - Timer - Gloves, gown, face shield
Standards	Required time = 70 minutes Performance time = _____ Total possible points = _____ Points earned = _____
Evaluation Rubric Codes: **S** = Satisfactory, meets standard **U** = Unsatisfactory, fails to meet standard	
NOTE: Steps marked with an ✱ are critical to achieve required competency.	

Preparation: Preanalytical Phase	Scores	
	S	**U**
A. Test information		
- Kit or instrument method **SEDIPLAST**		
- Manufacturer **Polymedco, Inc.**		
- Proper storage (temperature, light, etc.) **room temperature**		
- Lot number on package _____		
- Expiration date _____		
- Package insert or test flow chart available: _____ yes _____ no		
B. Personal protective equipment **gloves, gown, face shield**		
C. Proper specimen used for test		
- Type of specimen **fresh EDTA whole blood up to 2 hours or refrigerated blood up to 6 hours**		
- Specimen testing device **SEDIPLAST vial and pipette**		
D. Assembled all the above, sanitized hands, and applied personal protective equipment		
Procedure: Analytical Phase	**Scores**	
	S	**U**
E. Performed/observed quality control methods: not applicable		
F. Performed patient test	**S**	**U**
1. Removed stopper on vial and filled the vial with blood to indicated mark with a disposable transfer pipette (0.8 mL blood needed)		
2. Replaced vial stopper and inverted vial several times to mix		
3. Placed vial in SEDIPLAST rack on a level surface free of vibrations and jarring		

	S	U
4. Pressed the disposable SEDIPLAST pipette gently through the stopper with a twisting motion and continued to press until the pipette rested on the bottom of the vial (The pipette auto-zeros the blood and any excess flows into the closed reservoir compartment at the top of the pipette)		
5. Set the timer for 1 hour and let specimen stand undisturbed		
6. After 1 hour read the numeric results of the ESR (Use the scale at the top of the pipette to measure the distance from the top of the plasma to the top of the red blood cells.)		

*Accurate Results _____   Instructor Confirmation _____

Follow-up/Postanalytical Phase	Scores	
	S	U
*G. Proper documentation		
1. On patient log _____ yes _____ no		
2. Documented on patient chart (see below)		
3. Identified critical values and took appropriate steps to notify physician		
- ESR expected values: Men <50 years = 0 to 15 mm/hr Men > 50 years = 0 to 20 mm/hr Women <50 years = 0 to 20 mm/hr Women >50 years = 0 to 30 mm/hr		
H. Proper disposal and disinfection		
1. Disposed all sharps into biohazard sharps containers		
2. Disposed all other regulated medical waste into biohazard bags		
3. Disinfected test area and instruments according to OSHA guidelines		
4. Sanitized hands after removing gloves		
Totals Counts per Column		

Patient name: _____

Patient Chart Entry: (Don't forget to include when, what, why, any additional information, and the signature of the person charting.)

_____

_____

Analytical Test: ProTime Prothrombin Time

Person evaluated _____   Date _____

Evaluated by _____   Score/grade _____

Outcome goal	Perform FDA-approved prothrombin waived test following the most current OSHA safety guidelines and applying correct quality control
Conditions	Supplies needed:
	- ProTime cuvette - Tenderlett Plus (blood lancing and collection device) - Alcohol and gauze - Personal protective equipment
Standards	Required time = 10 minutes Performance time = _____ Total possible points = _____ Points earned = _____

Evaluation Rubric Codes:

S = Satisfactory, meets standard   **U** = Unsatisfactory, fails to meet standard

NOTE: Steps marked with an **✳** are critical to achieve required competency.

Preparation: Preanalytical Phase	Scores	
	S	**U**
A. Test information		
- Kit or instrument method **ProTime 3 Microcoagulation System**		
- Manufacturer **ITC ProTime 3**		
- Proper storage (temperature, light, etc.) **foil-pouched cuvette is refrigerated; once opened it must be used within 8 hours**		
- Expiration date _____		
- Lot number on cuvette _____		
- Package insert or test flow chart available: _____ yes _____ no		
B. Personal protective equipment **gloves, gown, face shield**		
C. Proper specimen used for test		
- Type of specimen **finger stick blood or plastic syringe blood**		
- Specimen container **Tenderlett Plus lancet and collection cup**		
D. Assembled all the above, sanitized hands, and applied personal protective equipment		
Procedure: Analytical Phase	Scores	
	S	**U**
E. Performed/observed quality control		
- Quantitative testing controls		
- Calibration check **ProTime instrument and cuvettes are precalibrated; no additional calibration is required**		
- Control levels **each test cuvette has three channels that run a level I control, a level II control, and the patient test simultaneously**		

F. Performed patient test	S	U
1. The fresh whole blood should pass the line on the Tenderlett collection cup		
2. Turned on ProTime		
- Pressed the "o" button		
- ProTime takes approximately 60 seconds to self-check (calibrate)		
- Waited for the next prompt		
3. Inserted test cuvette		
- The bar code should be face down		
- ProTime beeps when the cuvette is in place		
- ProTime warms the cuvette for 1 to 3 minutes		
4. Prepared the finger		
- Warmed hand to stimulate blood flow		
- Cleansed the finger with alcohol		
- Dried the finger thoroughly with gauze		
- Positioned Tenderlett and waited for the next prompt		
5. Incised the finger		
- Pinched Tenderlett Plus between the finger and thumb		
- Placed the other thumb over the red trigger		
- Pressed trigger		
6. Filled the cup to line		
- Wiped away the first drop		
- Formed a large drop of blood		
- Touched drop to cup		
- Kept adding blood until it passed the line on the cup		
7. Snapped Tenderlett Plus onto ProTime		
- Held the device at an angle		
- Placed cup end into slot		
- Pressed down to click in place		
8. Pressed the "o" button to start test		
- This signals ProTime to draw the sample from the cup into the cuvette. The screen will say "sampling"		
- Followed the instructions on screen: "Remove Tenderlett Plus"		
9. Removed Tenderlett Plus		
- Waited for the beep and the screen command to "Remove Tenderlett Plus"		
- *Important:* Removed the Tenderlett Plus immediately; ProTime allows 6 seconds. Failure to do so will result in a fault message.		
10. Read results		
- Recorded INR and prothrombin time.		
- Pressed the "o" button to turn off		
*Accurate Results INR = _____ PT = _____ Instructor Confirmation _____		

| Follow-up/Postanalytical Phase | Scores | |
	S	U
*G. Proper documentation		
1. On patient log _____ yes _____ no		
2. Documented on patient chart (see below)		

3. Identified critical values and took appropriate steps to notify physician
   ProTime expected values for both normal and therapeutic whole blood:

	INR	PT (in seconds) (ISI = 1.0)
Normal	0.8-1.2	10.4-15.7
Low anticoagulation	1.5-2.0	19.6-26.1
Moderate anticoagulation	2.0-3.0	26.1-39.2
High anticoagulation	2.5-4.0	32.6-52.2

H. Proper disposal and disinfection | |
1. Disposed all sharps into biohazard sharps containers
2. Disposed all other regulated medical waste into biohazard bags
3. Disinfected test area and instruments according to OSHA guidelines
4. Sanitized hands after removing gloves

Totals Counts per Column | |

Patient name: _____

Patient Chart Entry: (Don't forget to include when, what, why, any additional information, and the signature of the person charting.)

_____

_____

Skill Procedure: QBC Star Centrifugal Hematology System

Person evaluated _____   Date _____

Evaluated by _____   Score/grade _____

Outcome goal	Perform FDA-approved QBC Star moderately complex test following the most current OSHA safety guidelines and applying correct quality control
Conditions	Supplies required: - QBC Star tube (capillary) with cap - Lancet, alcohol, and gauze for capillary blood or EDTA Vacutainer tube and venipuncture supplies - Personal protective equipment
Standards	Required time = 10 minutes Performance time = _____ Total possible points = _____ Points earned = _____
Evaluation Rubric Codes:	
S = Satisfactory, meets standard **U** = Unsatisfactory, fails to meet standard	
NOTE: Steps marked with an ✱ are critical to achieve required competency.	

Preparation: Preanalytical Phase	Scores	
	S	U
A. Test information		
- Kit or instrument method **QBC Star hematology system**		
- Manufacturer **Becton Dickinson**		
- Proper storage (temperature, light, etc.) **QBC Star tubes, room temperature; liquid controls must be stored in refrigerator**		
- Expiration date _____		
- Lot number of QBC Star tubes _____		
- Package insert or test flow chart available _____ yes _____ no		
B. Personal protective equipment **gloves, gown, face shield, biohazard container**		
C. Specimen information		
- Type of specimen **capillary blood or whole blood from EDTA tube**		
- Specimen testing device **QBC Star tube (capillary tube system)**		
D. Assembled all the above, sanitized hands, and applied personal protective equipment		
Procedure: Analytical Phase	Scores	
	S	U
E. Performed/observed quantitative quality control		
- Calibration check instrument automatically calibrates itself and provides a printed readout each time it is turned on		
- Control levels level 1 and level 2 liquid controls must be run before testing patients with each new lot or newly received shipment of QBC Star tubes and at least monthly		
F. Performed patient test	S	U
1. Prepared the QBC Star tube		
- Blood source can be either a capillary finger stick drop of blood or anticoagulated venous blood from lavender-topped Vacutainer tube		

- Filled tube to second black fill line by capillary action		
- Did not allow the outer sleeve to come into contact with the blood		
- Wiped away blood on outside of tube		
2. Mixed the tube		
- Rocked the tube back and forth at least four times		
- Did not allow the blood to touch the pink plug at the end of the tube		
3. Tilted tube to bring blood toward the center of the tube		
4. Capped the tube		
- Removed cap from the tube by pulling it straight off (did not bend)		
- Placed the cap over the collection end of the tube by guiding the glass end of the tube into the center of the cap		
- Pushed cap on firmly, then pushed again while turning to seat the cap		
5. Inserted the tube into the instrument and closed the door		
- Placed tube with cap side up and the pink sealed end down		
- Closed the analyzer door, making sure it clicked into place		
6. Started the test by pressing the "Star" button		
- After mixing the specimen, the centrifuge accelerates to high speed to separate and pack the cell populations into distinct cell bands		
- A countdown displays the time remaining in the cycle		
- A series of messages and clicking sounds is seen and heard during the testing process		
- When the test is complete, the results are automatically displayed and printed.		

*Accurate Results _____   Instructor Confirmation _____

Follow-up/Postanalytical Phase	Scores	
	S	U
*G. Proper documentation		
1. On control log _____ yes _____ no		
2. On patient log _____ yes _____ no		
3. On patient chart (see below)		
4. Identified critical values and took appropriate steps to notify physician. Expected hematology ranges (adult):		

HCT (%) men	42-50
HCT (%) women	36-45
Hgb (g/dL) men	14-18
Hgb (g/dL) women	12-16
MCHC (g/dL)	31.7-36
PLT ($\times10^9$/L)	140-440
WBC ($\times10^9$/L)	4.3-10.0
Granulocytes ($\times10^9$/L)	1.8-7.2
Lymphocytes/monocytes ($\times10^9$/L)	1.7-4.9

H. Proper disposal and disinfection		
1. Disposed all sharps into biohazard sharps containers		
2. Disposed all other regulated medical waste into biohazard bags		
3. Disinfected test area and instruments according to OSHA guidelines		
4. Sanitized hands after removing gloves		
Totals Points per Column		

Patient Name: _____

Attach printed readout or write results below (circle result if outside range).

Test	Result	Reference Range
HCT (%) men		42-50
HCT (%) women		36-45
Hgb (g/dL) men		14-18
Hgb (g/dL) women		12-16
MCHC (g/dL)		31.7-36
PLT ($\times 10^9$/L)		140-440
WBC ($\times 10^9$/L)		4.3-10.0
Granulocytes ($\times 10^9$/L)		1.8-7.2
Lymphocytes/monocytes ($\times 10^9$/L)		1.7-4.9

Chemistry

VOCABULARY REVIEW

Match each fundamental term with the correct definition.

_____ 1. endogenous cholesterol

_____ 2. glycogen

_____ 3. exogenous cholesterol

_____ 4. catalysts

_____ 5. hyperinsulinemia

_____ 6. glycosylated Hgb

_____ 7. hyperlipidemia

_____ 8. insulin

_____ 9. glucagon

_____ 10. trans fats

_____ 11. ions

_____ 12. glycosuria

_____ 13. atherosclerosis

_____ 14. panels

_____ 15. dyslipidemia

_____ 16. carbohydrates

_____ 17. definitive diagnosis

_____ 18. hyperglycemia

_____ 19. clinical diagnosis

_____ 20. ketoacidosis

_____ 21. noncarbohydrate
energy sources

A. chemicals that produce specific changes in other substances without being changed themselves

B. groups of tests providing information on particular organs or body metabolism

C. glucose permanently changes the hemoglobin molecule within red blood cells

D. abnormal fat levels in the blood

E. formation of plaque along the inside walls of blood vessels

F. sugars and starches

G. sugar in the urine

H. cholesterol derived from the diet

I. manmade hydrogenated fats

J. elevated blood sugar

K. fats and proteins that are able to convert to glucose if necessary

L. electrolytes consisting of positively or negatively charged particles

M. excessively high blood insulin levels

N. hormone produced by the pancreas to lower blood glucose

O. diagnosis based on the patient's initial signs and symptoms

P. excessive fat in blood, giving a milky appearance in the plasma

Q. condition of excessive ketones in the blood causing an acid condition

R. hormone produced by the pancreas to raise blood glucose

S. stored form of glucose especially found in muscles and the liver

T. cholesterol manufactured in the liver

U. a final, confirmed diagnosis based on clinical signs and symptoms and the results of diagnostic tests

FUNDAMENTAL CONCEPTS

22. Provide the missing information in the plasma flow chart (refer to Figure 5-1).

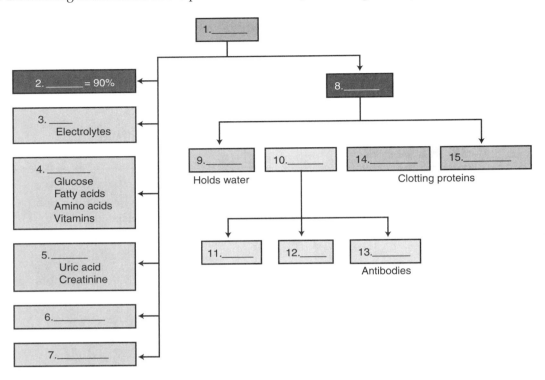

23. Match the following categories of chemicals found in plasma with their associated substances (refer to Figure 5-1).

___ clotting proteins

___ nutrients

___ hormones

___ proteins

___ wastes

___ salts

___ gamma globulins

___ enzymes

___ the three globulins

A. albumins and globulins

B. electrolytes

C. alpha, beta, and gamma

D. catalysts

E. glucose, amino acids, and fatty acids

F. antibodies

G. thyroid and pituitary glands

H. prothrombin and fibrinogen

I. urea, uric acid, creatinine

24. Describe the similarities and differences between the gold SST tube and the red SST tube.

_____

_____

_____

25. Refer to the sample requisition in the text (Figure 5-3) and identify what tube to use for each of the following tests:

    prothrombin time   _____   BUN   _____

    lipid panel   _____   CBC w/Diff   _____

    renal function panel   _____   mono test   _____

26. When prothrombin and fibrinogen are removed from plasma, the remaining liquid is referred to as _____.

27. Define the following glucose-related abbreviations.

    A1C   _____   IGT   _____

    FBG   _____   NIDDM   _____

    FPG   _____   OGTT   _____

    GTT   _____   2-hr PP   _____

    IDDM   _____

28. How is glucose metabolized in the following locations?

    body cells _____

    liver _____

    muscles _____

    adipose tissue _____

29. List the two ways insulin lowers blood glucose.

    _____

    _____

30. List the two ways glucagon raises blood glucose.

    _____

    _____

31. What are the two lifestyle changes a prediabetic patient can do to prevent or delay the development of type 2 diabetes?

    _____

    _____

32. List three beneficial functions of cholesterol.

    _____

    _____

33. List the two dietary fats that elevate the bad type of cholesterol (LDL).

    _____

    _____

34. Define the following lipid-related abbreviations.

HDL _____

LDL _____

TC/HDL ratio _____

VLDL _____

35. List two dietary fats that elevate the good type of cholesterol (HDL).

_____

_____

36. Why is LDL cholesterol referred to as "lousy" cholesterol and HDL referred to as "healthy" cholesterol?

_____

_____

37. Physicians are likely to be more interested in which of the following as a predictive indicator of possible future myocardial infarction?
    a. cholesterol value
    b. LDL value
    c. cholesterol/HDL ratio
    d. HDL value

38. People who exercise regularly, maintain normal weight, and eat mostly unsaturated fats will probably increase their level of
    a. HDL
    b. LDL
    c. albumin
    d. glucose

39. When testing for triglycerides, the patient should refrain from alcohol for ___ days before testing and fast for _____ hours before the test.

CLIA WAIVED CHEMISTRY TESTS

40. What is the purpose of calibrating a blood chemistry analyzer? (Hint: Think of the calibrator checks when running the Cholestech and the DCA 2000.)

_____

41. List three reasons or causes why a control would not fall within its designated range.

_____

_____

42. List three foods that should be avoided 2 days before collecting a fecal specimen used for the occult blood test.

_____

_____

43. List four drugs typically screened for in a urine specimen.

_____

_____

44. Label the DCA 2000 equipment and supplies (see Procedure 5-2 in textbook).

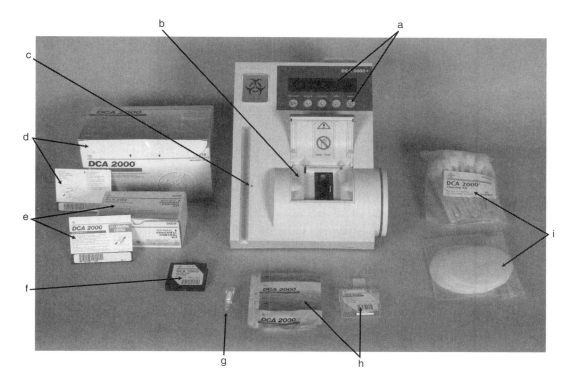

45. Label the Cholestech LDX equipment and supplies (see Procedure 5-3 in textbook).

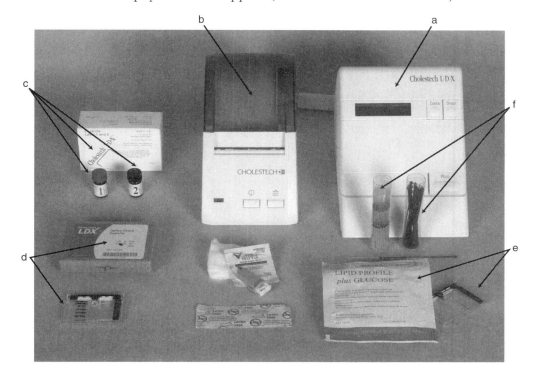

46. Label the ColoScreen III equipment and supplies (see Procedure 5-4 in textbook).

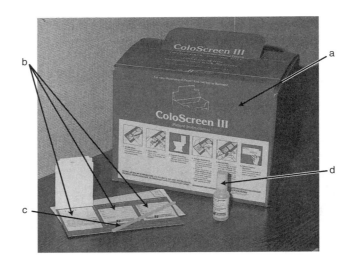

ADVANCED CONCEPTS

Match each procedural and advanced term with the correct definition.

_____ 47. cation

_____ 48. galvanometer

_____ 49. reflectance photometry

_____ 50. troponins I and T

_____ 51. bilirubin

_____ 52. absorbance photometry

_____ 53. anion

_____ 54. cannabinoid

_____ 55. transmittance photometry

_____ 56. calibration

_____ 57. occult

_____ 58. gout

_____ 59. opiates

_____ 60. myoglobin

A. form of arthritis caused by accumulation of uric acid crystals in the synovial fluid

B. hidden or not visible to the naked eye

C. heme-containing, oxygen-binding protein found in muscles

D. positively charged ion

E. "optics check" or setting to ensure the analyzer's optics are working correctly with the testing devices

F. measurement of the amount of light passing through the solution

G. methadone and morphine

H. heart-specific indicators of a recent myocardial infarction

I. measurement of the light that reflects off of the specimen

J. measurement of the amount of light the solution absorbs

K. waste product from the breakdown of hemoglobin

L. negatively charged ion

M. instrument capable of measuring the intensity of light

N. marijuana

61. Match the following panels with their representative group of tests.

_____ cardiac panel

_____ hepatic panel

_____ renal panel

_____ lipid panel

_____ thyroid panel

_____ metabolic panel

_____ electrolyte panel

A. 12 or more tests

B. BUN, creatinine, uric acid

C. sodium, potassium, chloride

D. bilirubin, AST, ALT, ALP, LD, GGT

E. troponins I and T, CK, LD, ALT, myoglobin

F. TSH, T4, T3 uptake

G. TC, HDL, LDL, triglycerides

62. Match the following analytes with the medical condition or organ that needs monitoring.

_____ uric acid   A. diabetes

_____ cholesterol   B. hepatitis or liver function

_____ BUN   C. gout

_____ glucose   D. coronary artery disease and atherosclerosis

_____ bilirubin   E. nephritis or kidney function

Chemistry Abbreviations

63. Using the alphabetical list of abbreviations at the front of Chapter 5 in the text, identify the six enzyme abbreviations routinely tested for tissue or organ damage. (Hint: remember enzymes have the suffix "-ase.") Then identify two organs or the diseases that are associated with each enzyme. Use the alphabetical chart of blood chemistry analytes (Table 5-3) at the end of the chapter to locate the diseases.

Enzyme Abbreviation	Enzyme	Affected Organs and Associated Diseases
1.		
2.		
3.		
4.		
5.		
6.		

64. List the four electrolyte abbreviations found at the beginning of the chapter and state whether they are cations or anions. (Hint: they will have positive or negative charges after their abbreviations.)

Electrolyte Abbreviation	Electrolyte	Cation/Anion $(+ / -)$
1.		
2.		
3.		
4.		

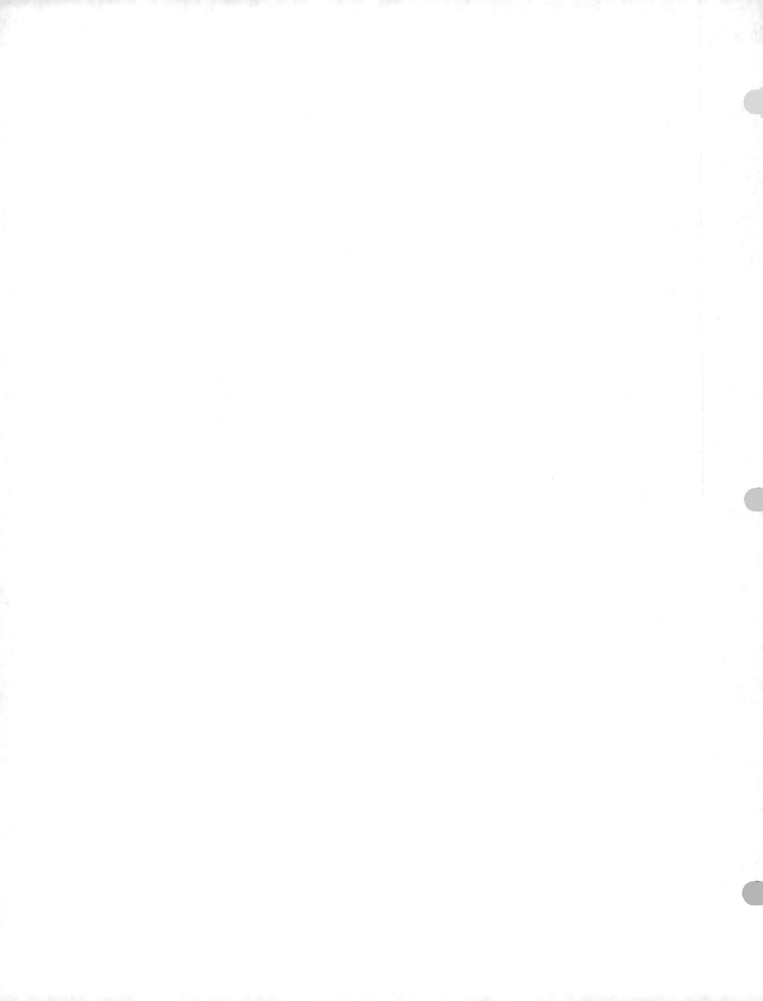

Analytical Test: Glucose—Glucometer

Person evaluated _____   Date _____

Evaluated by _____

Outcome goal	Perform FDA-approved CLIA waived glucose test following the most current OSHA safety guidelines and applying correct quality control
Conditions	Supplies needed: - Ascensia Elite or One Touch Test Strips - Coded test strip and liquid controls - Lancet, alcohol, gauze, bandage - Personal protective equipment
Standards	Required time = 5 minutes Performance time = _____ Total possible points = _____ Points earned = _____
Evaluation rubric codes **S** = Satisfactory, meets standard **U** = Unsatisfactory, fails to meet standard	
NOTE: Steps marked with an ***** are critical to achieve required competency.	

Preparation: Preanalytical Phase	Scores	
	S	**U**
A. Test information		
- Kit or instrument method **Ascensia Elite XL or One Touch Ultra**		
- Manufacturer **Bayer or LifeScan**		
- Proper storage (temperature, light, etc.) **foil-wrapped test strips and controls are stored at room temperature**		
- Expiration date _____		
- Lot # _____ Calibration # _____		
- Package insert or test flow chart available _____ yes _____ no		
B. Personal protective equipment - **gloves, gown, biohazard container**		
C. Specimen information		
- Type of specimen **fasting, 2-hour postprandial, or random specimen**		
- Specimen source **capillary blood**		
- Specimen testing device **coded test strips**		
D. Assembled all the above, sanitized hands, and applied personal protective equipment		

Procedure: Analytical Phase	Scores	
	S	**U**
E. Performed/observed quantitative quality control		
- Calibration check _____		
- (checked code number on meter against test strip number if needed)		
- Control levels: normal _____ high _____		
- (Manufacturer recommendation: run with each new batch of strips, with each new operator, then weekly)		
F. Performed patient test		
1. Turned on meter by inserting test strip's end with the contact bars		
2. Stuck finger and touched the end of the strip into the drop of blood, allowing the blood to flow ("sip") into the strip without interruption		
- Did **not** smear or place blood on top or bottom of strip		
3. When beep was heard, removed the glucometer and strip away from drop of blood		
4. Result displayed on the screen		

*Accurate Results _____   Instructor Confirmation _____

Follow-up/Postanalytical Phase	Scores	
	S	U
*G. Proper documentation		
1. On control log _____ yes _____ no		
2. On patient log _____ yes _____ no		
3. Documentation on patient chart (see below)		
H. Identified "critical values" and took appropriate steps to notify physician		

- Expected ranges for glucose based on ADA recommendations

		Fasting	2-hr Postprandial (After Drinking a Glucose-Rich Beverage)
	Normal	Less than 100 mg/dL	<140 mg/dL
	Prediabetes	100-125 mg/dL	140-199 mg/dL
	Diabetes	≥126 mg/dL	≥200 mg/dL

	Scores	
	S	U
I. Proper disposal and disinfection		
1. Disposed all sharps into biohazard sharps containers		
2. Disposed all other regulated medical waste into biohazard bags		
3. Disinfected test area and instruments according to OSHA guidelines		
4. Sanitized hands after removing gloves		
Total Points per Column		

Patient name: _____

Patient Chart Entry: (Don't forget to include when, what, how, why, any additional information, and the signature of the person charting.)

_____

_____

_____

_____

Analytical Test: Hemoglobin A1c—DCA 2000 Method

Person evaluated _____   Date _____

Evaluated by _____   Score/grade _____

Outcome goal	Perform FDA-approved glycosylated hemoglobin A1c waived test following the most current OSHA safety guidelines and applying the correct quality control
Conditions	Supplies needed: - Optical test cartridge (found in analyzer) - High and low liquid controls - Program cards for new test kits and liquid controls - Capillary tube holder and cartridge from test kit - Alcohol, gauze, and lancet or proper vacuum tube - Personal protective equipment
Standards	Required time = 10 minutes Performance time = _____ Total possible points = _____ Points earned = _____

Evaluation rubric codes:
S = Satisfactory, meets standard   **U** = Unsatisfactory, fails to meet standard

NOTE: Steps marked with an * are critical to achieve required competency.

Preparation: Preanalytical Phase	Scores	
	S	**U**
A. Test information		
- Kit or instrument method **DCA 2000+ Analyzer**		
- Manufacturer Bayer		
- Proper storage (temperature, light, etc.) **Foil-wrapped cartridges are refrigerated. Allow 10 minutes for the refrigerated, wrapped cartridge to warm to room temperature. If refrigerated cartridge is removed from wrap, it can be used in 5 minutes but must then be used within 1 hour.**		
- Expiration date _____		
- Lot # of cartridges _____		
- Package insert or test flow chart available _____ yes _____ no		
B. Personal protective equipment **gloves, gown, face shield**		
C. Proper specimen used for test		
- Type of specimen: fresh capillary blood or whole blood from EDTA, heparin, citrate and/or fluoride/oxalate only (do not use any other anticoagulants). Can also use venous whole blood that has been refrigerated within 1 week of collection (be sure it is well mixed and warmed to room temperature).		
- Specimen testing device: microcapillary tube provided in kit		
D. Assembled all the above, sanitized hands, and applied personal protective equipment		

Procedure: Analytical Phase	Scores	
	S	**U**
E. Performed/observed quantitative quality control		
- Optics check: scanned black cartridge and then placed cartridge into test compartment. Checked results against reference range.		
- Control levels: normal _____ abnormal _____		
- Calibration scanning cards must be scanned before running controls. Follow manufacturer's recommendations on control monitoring.		

	S	U
F. Performed patient test		
1. Touched tip of capillary into drop of blood until capillary was filled		
- The blood should fill the small glass capillary tube without touching the plastic holder		
- Once glass capillary is filled with sample, analysis must begin within 5 minutes		
2. Wiped sides of capillary tube with tissue		
3. Inserted capillary holder into cartridge (flat side toward cartridge) until holder snapped into place		
4. Scanned cartridge through bar code reader on left side of analyzer		
- Held cartridge so that bar code faced right		
- Inserted cartridge into bar code track above dot and slid down quickly		
- A beep and display change indicated a successful scan; repeated scan if not successful		
5. Inserted cartridge into test compartment until a click was heard		
- Held cartridge so that bar code faced right		
6. Slowly and firmly pulled to remove pull tab while holding down cartridge		
7. Closed door		
8. After test was completed, recorded results from display and reported to physician		
9. Removed cartridge		
- Held button on right side of compartment down with right hand		
- Left hand gently pushed plastic tab on cartridge to the right to unlock.		
- Pulled upward to remove cartridge from compartment		

* **Accurate Results** _____ **Instructor Confirmation** _____

Follow-up/Postanalytical Phase	Scores	
	S	U
* G. Proper documentation		
1. Control logs _____ yes _____ no		
2. Patient log _____ yes _____ no		
3. Documented on patient chart (see below)		
4. Identified critical values and took appropriate steps to notify physician		
- Expected values:		

Nondiabetics	3%-6%
Controlled diabetics	6%-8%
Poorly controlled diabetics	As much as 20% or higher
(Normal ranges should be determined by each laboratory to conform with the population being tested)	

	S	U
H. Proper disposal and disinfection		
1. Disposed all sharps into biohazard sharps containers		
2. Disposed all other regulated medical waste into biohazard bags		
3. Disinfected test area and instruments according to OSHA guidelines		
4. Sanitized hands after removing gloves		
Total Points per Column:		

Patient name: _____

Patient Chart Entry: (Don't forget to include when, what, how, why, any additional information, and the signature of the person charting.)

_____

_____

_____

Analytical Test: Lipid Profile—Cholestech Method

Person evaluated _____   Date _____

Evaluated by _____

Outcome goal	Perform FDA-approved Lipid Profile waived test following the most current OSHA safety guidelines and applying the correct quality control.
Conditions	Supplies needed: - Optics check cassette - Level 1 and 2 liquid controls - Alcohol, gauze and lancets or vacuum lithium heparin tubes - Capillary tubes and plungers for finger stick sample - Mini-Pet Pipette and Pipette Tips for venipuncture sample - Personal protective equipment
Standards	Required time = 10 minutes Performance time = _____ Total possible points = _____ Points earned _____

Evaluation rubric codes:
S = Satisfactory, meets standard   **U** = Unsatisfactory, fails to meet standard

NOTE: Steps marked with an * are critical to achieve required competency.

Preparation: Preanalytical Phase	Scores	
	S	U
A. Test information		
- Kit or instrument method Cholestech LDX Analyzer		
- Manufacturer **Cholestech Corporation**		
- Proper storage (temperature, light, etc.) **foil-wrapped cassettes are refrigerated. They must return to room temperature before testing.**		
- Expiration date _____		
- Cassette lot # _____		
- Package insert or test flow chart available _____ yes _____ no		
B. Personal protective equipment **gloves, gown, biohazard containers**		
C. Specimen Information		
- Patient preparation **Cholesterol recommends fasting. Triglyceride requires fasting and no alcohol consumption in previous 48 hours.**		
- Type of specimen **capillary blood or lithium heparin (green) tube only for venous blood**		
- Specimen testing **device Cholestech capillary tube (once in tube, must be tested within 5 minutes)**		
D. Assembled all the above, sanitized hands, and applied personal protective equipment		
Procedure: Analytical Phase	Scores	
	S	U
E. Performed/observed quantitative quality control		
- Calibration check (**run calibration cassette daily**)		
- Control levels **Level 1, Level 2** (Use the mini-Pet pipettes provided by Cholestech)		
F. Performed patient test	S	U
1. Allowed cassette to come to room temperature (at least 10 minutes before opening)		
2. Made sure analyzer was plugged in and warmed up		

3. Removed cassette from its pouch and placed it on flat surface		
- Held cassette by the short sides only		
- Did not touch the black bar or the brown magnetic strip		
4. Pressed RUN; the analyzer did a self-test and the screen displayed: "selftest running" and then "selftest OK"		
5. The cassette drawer opened and the screen displayed: "load cassette and press RUN"		
- Drawer will remain open for 4 minutes, after which it will close with the message "System timeout: RUN to continue." If the RUN button is not pushed within 15 seconds, the drawer will close and the screen will go blank. Press RUN again, allow to go through the self-test again, then proceed.		
6. Collected fresh capillary blood to the black line of the capillary tube with plunger inserted into the red end of the tube		
- Or, collected fresh venous whole blood with the Cholestech mini-Pet pipette		
7. Placed whole blood sample into the test cassette sample well		
- The fingerstick sample must be put into the cassette within 5 minutes of collection or the blood will clot		
8. *Immediately* placed cassette into the drawer of the Analyzer		
- Kept cassette level after the sample was applied		
- The black reaction bar faced toward the analyzer		
- The brown magnetic strip was on the right		
9. Pressed RUN. The drawer closed and the screen displayed: "[test names] - running"		
10. When the test was completed, the Analyzer beeped and the screen displayed results at the same time the printer printed out results. (Press DATA to display the calculated results of all tests on the screen if running a panel of tests.)		

* **Accurate Results** _____   **Instructor Confirmation** _____

	Scores	
Follow-up/Postanalytical Phase	**S**	**U**
* G. Proper documentation		
1. On control log _____ yes _____ no		
2. On patient log _____ yes _____ no		
3. Documented on patient chart (see below)		
4. Identified "critical values" and took appropriate steps to notify physician		
- NCEP ATP III guidelines for lipid panels:		

Test	Desirable
Total cholesterol (TC)	<200 mg/dL
HDL cholesterol	>40 mg/dL
LDL cholesterol	<130 mg/dL
Triglycerides	<150 mg/dL
TC/HDL ratio	≤4.5
Glucose	Fasting: 60-110 mg/dL
	Nonfasting: <less than 160 mg/dL
Alanine aminotransferase	10-40 U/L

H. Proper disposal and disinfection		
1. Disposed all sharps into biohazard sharps containers		
2. Disposed all other regulated medical waste into biohazard bags		
3. Disinfected test area and instruments according to OSHA guidelines		
4. Sanitized hands after removing gloves		
Total Points per Column		

Patient name: _____

Attach printed readout or record results below:

Test	Results	Desirable
Total cholesterol (TC)		<200 mg/dL
HDL cholesterol		> 40 mg/dL
LDL cholesterol		<130 mg/dL
Triglycerides		<150 mg/dL
TC/HDL ratio		≤4.5
Glucose		Fasting: 60-110 mg/dL
		Nonfasting: <160 mg/dL

Analytical Test: Fecal Occult Blood—ColoScreen III Method

Person evaluated _____   Date _____

Evaluated by _____   Score/grade _____

Outcome goal	Perform FDA-approved CLIA waived fecal occult blood test following the most current OSHA safety guidelines and applying the correct quality control
Conditions	Supplies required: - Three specimen slides - Three wooden applicators - Hydrogen peroxide developer - Personal protective equipment
Standards	Required time = 5 minutes Performance time = _____ Total possible points = _____ Points earned = _____
Evaluation rubric codes: **S** = Satisfactory, meets standard	**U** = Unsatisfactory, fails to meet standard
NOTE: Steps marked with an * are critical to achieve required competency.	

Preparation: Preanalytical Phase	Scores	
	S	**U**
A. Test information		
- Kit or instrument method **ColoScreen III**		
- Manufacturer **SmithKline Diagnostics**		
- Proper storage (temperature, light, etc.) **room temperature**		
- Expiration date _____		
- Lot # on kit _____		
- Package insert or test flow chart available _____ yes _____ no		
B. Instructed patient on the following dietary preparations		
1. Two days before the test and during testing time, the patient should eat a high-fiber diet with any of the following:		
- Well-cooked poultry and fish		
- Cooked fruits and vegetables		
- Bran cereals		
- Raw lettuce, carrots, and celery		
- Moderate amounts of peanuts and popcorn		
2. The patient should avoid ingesting the following substances, which will interfere with the test results:		
- Red and partially cooked meats		
- Turnips, cauliflower, broccoli, parsnips, and melons (especially cantaloupe)		
- Alcohol, aspirin, and vitamin C		
C. Instructed the patient on how to use the slides, applicators, and the take-home instructions as follows:		
- After a bowel movement use the wooden applicator and collect a small sample of feces and spread a thin layer in box A of the slide		
- Using the same applicator, collect a second sample from an different part of the feces and spread it in box B		
- Discard the wooden applicator and reseal the cover of the slide and complete the information requested on the outside of the cover		
- Repeat the above with the remaining applicators with the next two bowel movements and two remaining slides		

Procedure: Analytical Phase	Scores	
	S	U
D. Personal protective equipment gloves when testing the slides		
E. Performed occult blood test as follows:		
- Confirmed all necessary information was written on slide covers		
- Applied gloves and observed universal precautions		
- Opened the back sides of all three slides and placed two drops of developer on each specimen		
- Observed slide for 30 seconds to 2 minutes and checked to see if a blue reaction occurred, indicating a positive result		
F. Performed monitor test (internal control)		
- Placed one or two drops between the monitor boxes and observed for 30 seconds to 2 minutes to read the results		
- Confirmed the positive turned blue and the negative did not		
* Accurate Results _____ Instructor Confirmation _____		

Follow-up/Postanalytical Phase	Scores	
	S	U
* G. Proper documentation		
1. On control/patient log _____ yes _____ no		
2. Documented on patient chart (see below)		
3. Identified critical values and took appropriate steps to notify physician		
- Expected values for occult blood: negative		
H. Proper disposal and disinfection		
- Disposed all regulated medical waste into biohazard bags		
- Disinfected test area and instruments according to OSHA guidelines		
- Sanitized hands after removing gloves		
Total Points per Column		

Patient name: _____

Patient Chart Entry: (Don't forget to include when, what, how, why, any additional information, and the signature of the person charting.)

_____

_____

_____

_____

Immunology

VOCABULARY REVIEW

Match the each term with its correct definition.

A. active immunity   G. histamine   M. normal flora

B. autoimmune diseases   H. humoral immunity   N. passive immunity

C. antibodies   I. inflammation   O. phagocytes

D. antigens   J. interferons   P. phagocytosis

E. cell-mediated immunity   K. mucous membrane

F. complement proteins   L. natural killer cells

_____ 1. B lymphocytic cell response to antigens resulting in the production of specific antibodies to destroy a foreign invader; also called antibody-mediated immunity

_____ 2. Cells capable of engulfing and ingesting microorganisms and cellular debris

_____ 3. Compound released by injured cells that causes the dilation of blood vessels

_____ 4. Immunoglobulins produced specifically to destroy foreign invaders

_____ 5. Long-term protection against future infections resulting from the production of antibodies formed naturally during an infection or artificially by vaccination

_____ 6. Nonpathogenic microorganisms that normally inhabit the skin and mucous membranes

_____ 7. Overall reaction of the body to tissue injury or invasion by an infectious agent; characterized by redness, heat, swelling, and pain

_____ 8. Process of engulfing and digesting microorganisms and cellular debris

_____ 9. Proteins secreted by infected cells to prevent the further replication and spread of an infection into neighboring cells

_____ 10. Proteins that stimulate phagocytosis and inflammation and are capable of destroying bacteria

_____ 11. Short-term acquired immunity created by antibodies received naturally through the placenta (or the colostrum to an infant) or artificially by injection

_____ 12. Special type of lymphocyte that attacks and destroys infected cells and cancer cells in a nonspecific way

____ 13. Substances that are perceived as foreign to the body and elicit an antibody response

____ 14. T-lymphocytic cell response to antigens

____ 15. Thin sheets of tissue that line the internal cavities and canals of the body and serve as a barrier against the entry of pathogens

____ 16. Destructive tissue diseases caused by antibody/self-antigen reactions

Match the following B and T lymphocytes with their functions.

A. killer T cells   D. helper T cells (TH4 or CD4)

B. suppressor T cells   E. memory B cells

C. plasma cells   F. memory T cells

____ 17. Antigen-activated B lymphocytes that remember an identified antigen for future encounters

____ 18. Antigen-activated lymphocytes that attack foreign antigens directly and destroy cells that bear the antigens; also called cytotoxic cells

____ 19. Antigen-activated lymphocytes that inhibit T and B cells after enough cells have been activated

____ 20. Antigen-activated lymphocytes that stimulate other T cells and help B cells produce antibodies

____ 21. Antigen-activated T lymphocytes that remember an antigen for future encounters

____ 22. Subgroup of B lymphocytes that produce the antibodies that travel through the blood specifically targeting and reacting with antigens

Match the following immunology testing and disease terms with the correct definition.

A. agglutination   E. immunosorbent   I. serology

B. chromatographic   F. in vitro   J. titer

C. erythroblastosis fetalis   G. in vivo   K. vaccination

D. heterophile antibody   H. self-antigens   L. wheal

____ 23. Antibody that appears during an Epstein-Barr viral infection (mononucleosis) that has an unusual affinity to heterophile antigens on sheep red cells

____ 24. Branch of laboratory medicine that performs antibody/antigen testing with serum

____ 25. Clumping together of blood cells or latex beads caused by antibodies adhering to their antigens

____ 26. A hemolytic anemia in newborns resulting from maternal-fetal blood group incompatibility

____ 27. Testing in a laboratory apparatus

____ 28. Pertaining to a visual color change that appears when an enzyme-linked antibody/antigen reaction occurs

____ 29. Pertaining to the attachment of an antigen or antibody to a solid surface such as latex beads, wells in plastic dishes, or plastic cartridges

____ 30. Process of injecting harmless or killed microorganisms into the body to induce immunity against a potential pathogen (also called immunization)

____ 31. Raised induration

____ 32. Substances within the body that induce the production of antibodies that attack an individual's own body tissues; also called auto-antigens

____ 33. A quantitative test that measures the amount of antibody that reacts with a specific antigen

____ 34. Testing within a host or living organism

FUNDAMENTAL CONCEPTS

35. When a pathogen is invading the body, list *two* examples of protection at each of the following lines of defense:

    First line of external defenses: _____

    Second line of internal, nonspecific defenses: _____

    _____

    Third line of internal, specific defenses: _____

    _____

36. List two white cells that are phagocytic.

    _____

37. Give an example of a normal flora organism and describe how it prevents the invasion of pathogens.

    _____

    _____

38. List the clinical signs of inflammation.

    _____

39. Describe antigens.

    _____

    _____

40. Which cells are associated with cell-mediated immunity?

    _____

41. What is another name for antibodies? (Hint: They are a subcategory of proteins.)

    _____

42. Name the five types of antibodies by their immunoglobulin identification.

    _____

43. Refer to Figure 6-4, *A* and *B* in the text and give examples of natural and artificial active immunity and natural and artificial passive immunity.

_____

_____

CLIA WAIVED IMMUNOLOGY TESTS

44. The pregnancy test determines the presence of what antigenic substance?

_____

_____

45. Fill in the blanks for the following medical information regarding infectious mononucleosis:

Causative agent: _____

Clinical symptoms: _____

Hematology findings: _____

Immunology findings: _____

46. Label the QuickVue+ infectious mononucleosis supplies (see Procedure 6-2 in textbook).

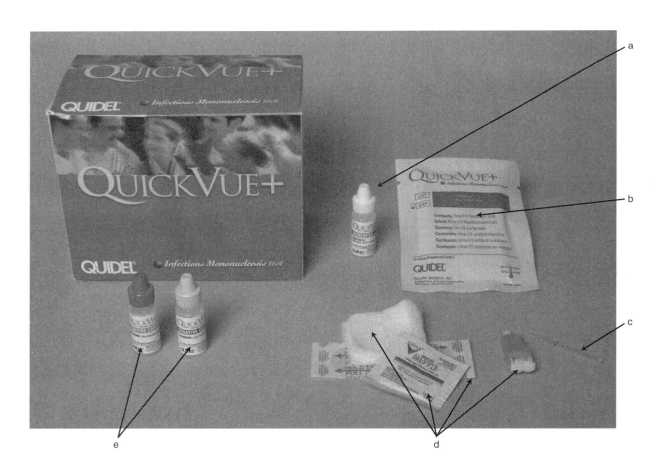

47. Describe the relation between *Helicobacter pylori* and ulcers.

_____

_____

48. Label the QuickVue *H. pylori* supplies (see Procedure 6-3 in textbook).

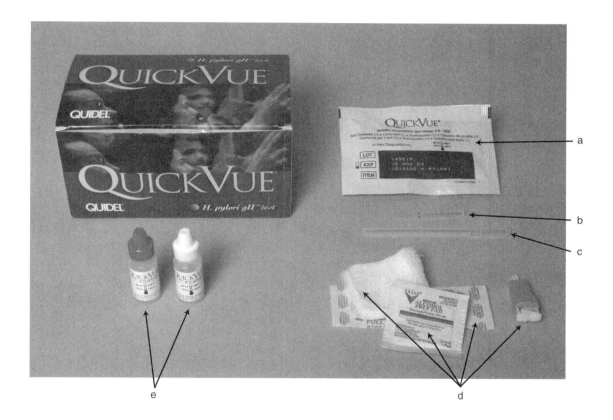

49. Define immunohematology and give three reasons why testing is done in this area.

_____

_____

50. Based on the test results pictured in the chart below, interpret the results for each test as either negative, positive, or invalid.

	Test	Figure in Text	Interpreted Result
A		Figure 6-6	_____
B		Procedure 6-1, *B*	_____
C		Procedure 6-2, *D*	_____

ADVANCED CONCEPTS

51. Define agglutination.

_____

_____

52. Give the blood type for a person who has the following: A and D antigens on red blood cells and anti-B antibodies in the serum.

_____

53. Give the antigens and antibodies present in type AB blood.

_____

54. Identify the following ABO blood types based on their agglutination reactions with anti-A and anti-B sera. (Hint: see Procedure 6-3 in the text.)

Blood Type	Reaction with Anti-A and Anti-B	
	Anti-A serum	Anti-B serum
_____		
_____		
_____		
_____		

55. Identify which of the following is Rh positive and which is Rh negative. (Hint: see Procedure 6-4 in the text.)

Rh Type	Reaction with Rh (anti-D) on the Left and the Negative Control on the Right
_____	
_____	

56. When the body is exposed to the following pathogens, it produces specific antibodies that can be measured in the plasma or serum. Refer to Table 6-3 in the text and identify the following pathogenic diseases and whether the pathogen is a bacteria or virus.

Pathogen	Disease	Bacteria or Virus
RSV		
Rubella		
Chlamydia		
Varicella zoster		
B. burgdorferi		

57. List three cancers that can be detected by immunologic testing (see Table 6-3 in the text).

_____

_____

Analytical Test: Urine Pregnancy—SureStep Method

Person evaluated _____   Date _____

Evaluated by _____   Score/Grade _____

Outcome goal	Perform FDA-approved CLIA waived urine pregnancy test following the most current OSHA safety guidelines and applying the correct quality control

Conditions	Supplies required:
	- SureStep test kit containing:
	  - Individually wrapped test devices
	  - Disposal dropper pipettes
	  - Instruction insert
	- Other materials needed
	- Urine collection container
	- Timer
	- Liquid positive and negative controls for human chorionic gonadotropin (hCG)

Standards	Required time = 5 minutes Performance time = _____ Total possible points = _____ Points earned = _____

Evaluation rubric codes:
S = Satisfactory, meets standard   **U** = Unsatisfactory, fails to meet standard

NOTE: Steps marked with an ***** are critical to achieve required competency.

SureStep Pregnancy Test		
Preparation: Preanalytical Phase	**Scores**	
	S	U
A. Test information		
- Kit method **SureStep**		
- Manufacturer **Applied Biotech, Inc.**		
- Proper storage (temperature, light, etc.) **refrigerator or room temperature**		
- Lot # of kit _____		
- Expiration date _____		
- Package insert or test flow chart available _____ yes _____ no		
B. Personal protective equipment **gloves, gown, biohazard container**		
C. Specimen information **clear urine specimen (centrifuge if cloudy)**		
- Type of specimen **Preferably first morning urine specimen. Urine can be stored in refrigerator for up to 72 hours but must be tested at room temperature.**		
- Appropriate container **clean, dry plastic or glass container**		
Procedure for SureStep hCG: Analytical Phase	**Scores**	
	S	U
D. Performed/observed qualitative quality control		
- External liquid controls positive _____ negative _____		
- Internal control: **a colored band will appear in the control region (C)**		
E. Performed patient test	S	U
1. Sanitized hands and applied gloves		
2. Removed test device from its protective pouch and labeled with patient identification		
- Brought to room temperature before opening to avoid condensation		

	S	U
3. Drew up the urine sample to the line marked on the pipette provided in kit		
- Approximately 0.2 mL		
- Used separate pipettes and devices for each specimen and control		
4. Dispensed entire contents into the sample well		
5. Waited for pink-colored bands to appear		
- High concentrations of hCG can be observed in as little as 40 seconds		
- Low concentrations may need 4 minutes for reaction time		
- Did not interpret results after 10 minutes		
6. At 5 minutes read and recorded the results (circle result)		
- Positive = two distinct pink bands appear, one in the patient test region (T) and one in the control region (C)		
- Negative = only one pink band appears in the control region (C); no apparent pink band appears in the patient test region (T)		
- Invalid = a total absence of pink bands in control region; test must be repeated with a new device. If problem persists called for assistance.		

* Accurate Results _____   Instructor Confirmation _____

Follow-up/Postanalytical	Scores	
	S	U
* F. Proper documentation		
1. On control/patient log _____ yes _____ no		
2. Documented on patient chart (see below)		
3. Identified critical values and took appropriate steps to notify physician		
- Expected values for analyte: negative for pregnancy		
G. Proper disposal and disinfection		
1. Disposed all sharps into biohazard sharps containers		
2. Disposed all other regulated medical waste into biohazard bags		
3. Disinfected test area and instruments according to OSHA guidelines		
Total Points per Column		

Patient name: _____

Patient Chart Entry: (Don't forget to include when, what, how, why, any additional information, and the signature of the person charting.)

_____

_____

_____

Analytical Test: Infectious Mononucleosis Test—QuickVue Method

Person evaluated _____   Date _____

Evaluated by _____   Score/Grade _____

Outcome goal	Perform FDA-approved CLIA waived infectious mononucleosis test following the most current OSHA safety guidelines and applying the correct quality control

Conditions	Supplies required:
	- QuickVue test kit containing:
	  - Developer
	  - Individually wrapped reaction units
	  - Capillary tubes for capillary blood and pipettes for venous blood
	  - Positive and negative liquid controls
	  - Instruction insert and pictorial flow chart
	- Other materials needed
	- Capillary puncture supplies (lancet, alcohol, gauze, bandage), or
	- whole blood venipuncture specimen
	- Timer
	- Personal protective equipment

Standards	Required time = 10 minutes Performance time = _____ Total possible points = _____ Points earned = _____
Evaluation rubric codes: **S** = Satisfactory, meets standard **U** = Unsatisfactory, fails to meet standard	
NOTE: Steps marked with an * are critical to achieve required competency.	

Preparation for Mononucleosis Test: Preanalytical Phase	Scores S	Scores U
A. Test information		
- Kit method **QuickVue+ Mononucleosis Test**		
- Manufacturer **Quidel**		
- Proper storage (temperature, light, etc.) **room temperature**		
- Lot # of kit _____		
- Expiration date _____		
- Package insert or test flow chart available _____ yes _____ no		
B. Personal protective equipment gloves, gown, biohazard containers		
C. Specimen information		
- Use the capillary transfer tube provided in the kit to obtain capillary blood or the larger transfer pipette in the kit to obtain the venipuncture whole blood, and the liquid controls.		
Procedure for Mononucleosis: Analytical Phase	**S**	**U**
D. Performed/observed qualitative quality control		
- External liquid controls positive _____ negative _____		
- Internal control **the color blue fills the "read result" window**		
E. Performed patient test	**S**	**U**
1. Dispensed all the blood from the capillary tube into the "add" well or transferred a large drop from the venous whole blood specimen with the pipette		
2. Added five drops of developer to the "add" well		
- Held bottle vertical and allowed drops to fall freely		

	S	U
3. Read results at 5 minutes		
- "test complete" line must be visible by 10 minutes		
4. Interpretation of results (circled result):		
- Positive = Any shade of a blue vertical line forms (+) sign in the "read result" window along with the blue "test complete" line. Even a faint blue vertical line should be reported as a positive result.		
- Negative = No blue vertical line in the "read result" window along with the blue "test complete" line.		
- Invalid = after 10 minutes no signal is observed in the "test complete" window, or the color blue fills the "read result" window. If either of these occurs, the test must be repeated with a new reaction unit. If the problem continues, contact technical support.		

* **Accurate Results** _____   **Instructor Confirmation** _____

	Scores	
Follow-up/Postanalytical Phase	**S**	**U**
* F. Proper documentation		
1. On control/patient log _____ yes _____ no		
2. Documented on patient chart (see below)		
3. Identified critical values and took appropriate steps to notify physician		
- Expected values for analyte: negative for mononucleosis		
G. Proper disposal and disinfection		
1. Disposed all sharps into biohazard sharps containers		
2. Disposed all other regulated medical waste into biohazard bags		
3. Disinfected test area and instruments according to OSHA guidelines		
4. Sanitized hands after removing gloves		
Total Points per Column		

Patient name: _____

Patient Chart Entry: (Don't forget to include when, what, how, why, any additional information, and the signature of the person charting.)

_____

_____

_____

Analytical Test: *Helicobacter pylori*—QuickVue Method

Person evaluated _____   Date _____

Evaluated by _____   Score/Grade _____

Outcome goal	Perform a CLIA waived *H. pylori* test following the most current OSHA safety guidelines and applying the correct quality controls

Conditions	Supplies required:
	- QuickVue *H. Pylori* test kit containing:
	  - Foil-wrapped test cassettes
	  - Plastic capillary tubes for fingerstick blood
	  - Disposable droppers for venous blood
	  - Liquid controls: positive and negative external controls
	  - Direction insert and procedure card
	- Other materials needed:
	  - Capillary puncture supplies (lancet, alcohol, gauze, bandage), or whole blood venipuncture specimen
	  - Timer
	  - Personal protective equipment

Standards	Required time = 10 minutes Performance time = _____ Total possible points = _____ Points earned = _____
Evaluation rubric codes: **S** = Satisfactory, meets standard; **U** = unsatisfactory, fails to meet standard	
NOTE: Steps marked with an ***** are critical to achieve required competency.	

Preparation for *H. pylori* Test: Preanalytical Phase	Scores	
	S	**U**
A. Test information		
- Kit method **QuickVue *H. pylori* gII test**		
- Manufacturer **Quidel**		
- Proper storage of kit: **room temperature**		
- Lot # of kit _____		
- Expiration date _____		
- Package insert or test flow chart available _____ yes _____ no		
B. Personal protective equipment **gloves, gown, biohazard containers**		
C. Specimen information		
- Use the capillary tube provided in the kit to obtain capillary blood or the larger disposable dropper in the kit to obtain the venipuncture whole blood specimen, and the liquid controls.		
Procedure for *H. pylori*: Analytical Phase	Scores	
	S	**U**
D. Performed/observed qualitative quality control		
- External liquid controls: positive _____ negative _____		
- Internal control **a blue band of color near the letter "C"**		
E. Performed patient test	**S**	**U**
1. Dispensed the blood into the sample well by one of the following methods:		
- Transferred a large drop from the venous anticoagulated whole blood specimen with the disposable dropper		

- Dispensed all the fingerstick blood from the capillary tube		
- Added two hanging drops of whole blood directly from a fingerstick into the round sample well on the test cassette		
2. Read and recorded results at 5 minutes		
- Did not move the test cassette until the assay was complete		
- Some positive results may be seen earlier than 5 minutes		
3. Interpretation of results (circle result)		
- Positive = a pink line next to the letter T and a blue line next to the letter C		
- Negative = only a blue line next to the letter C		
- Invalid = no blue line next to the letter C; the test must be repeated with a new cassette. If the problem continues, contact technical support.		

* **Accurate Results** _____ **Instructor Confirmation** _____

Follow-up/Postanalytical	Scores	
	S	U
* F. Proper documentation		
1. On control/patient log _____ yes _____ no		
2. Documented on patient chart (see below)		
3. Identified critical values and took appropriate steps to notify physician		
- Expected values for analyte: negative for *H. pylori*		
G. Proper disposal and disinfection		
1. Disposed all sharps into biohazard sharps containers		
2. Disposed all other regulated medical waste into biohazard bags		
3. Disinfected test area and instruments according to OSHA guidelines		
4. Sanitized hands after removing gloves		
Total Points per Column		

Patient name: _____

Patient Chart Entry: (Don't forget to include when, what, how, why, any additional information, and the signature of the person charting.)

_____

_____

_____

Analytical Test

Qualitative Test: _____

Person evaluated _____   Date _____

Evaluated by _____   Score/Grade _____

Outcome goal	
Conditions	Supplies required:
Standards	Required time = _____ Performance time = _____ Total possible points = _____ Points earned = _____
Evaluation rubric codes: **S** = Satisfactory, meets standard **U** = Unsatisfactory, fails to meet standard	
NOTE: Steps marked with an ***** are critical to achieve required competency.	

Preparation: Preanalytical Phase	Scores	
	S	U
A. Test information		
- Kit method		
- Manufacturer		
- Proper storage (temperature, light, etc.)		
- Lot # of kit _____		
- Expiration date _____		
- Package insert or test flow chart available: _____yes _____ no		
B. Personal protective equipment		
C. Specimen information		

Procedure: Analytical Phase	Scores	
	S	U
D. Performed/observed qualitative quality control		
- External liquid controls: positive _____ negative _____		
- Internal control		
E. Performed patient test		
1.		
2.		
3.		
4.		
Positive =		
Negative =		
Invalid =		
* Accurate Results _____ Instructor Confirmation _____		

Follow-up/Postanalytical Phase	Scores	
	S	U
*F. Proper documentation		
1. On control/patient log _____ yes _____ no		
2. Documentation on patient chart (see below)		
3. Identified critical values and took appropriate steps to notify physician		
- Expected values for analyte:		
G. Proper disposal and disinfection		
1. Disposed all sharps into biohazard sharps containers		
2. Disposed all other regulated medical waste into biohazard bags		
3. Disinfected test area and instruments according to OSHA guidelines		
4. Sanitized hands after removing gloves		
Total Points per Column		

Patient name: _____

Patient Chart Entry: (Don't forget to include when, what, how, why, any additional information, and the signature of the person charting.)

_____

_____

_____

CHAPTER 7

Microbiology

VOCABULARY REVIEW

_____ 1. malaise

_____ 2. myalgia

_____ 3. expectoration

_____ 4. gram-positive

_____ 5. fastidious

_____ 6. mortality

_____ 7. gram-negative

_____ 8. infection

_____ 9. peptidoglycan

_____ 10. morbidity

_____ 11. eukaryotic

_____ 12. prokaryote

_____ 13. binary fission

A. Rate at which illness occurs

B. Having the pink/red color of the counterstain used in Gram's method of staining microorganisms

C. Diffuse muscle pain

D. Pertaining to unicellular organisms that do not have a true nucleus with a nuclear membrane

E. Retaining the purple color of the stain used in Gram's method of staining microorganisms

F. Disease in the body caused by the invasion of pathogenic microorganisms

G. Coughing up sputum and mucus from the trachea and lungs

H. Component made of polysaccharides and peptides that gives rigidity to the bacterial cell wall

I. Feeling of weakness, distress, or discomfort

J. Requiring special nutrients for growth

K. Pertaining to organisms that possess a true nucleus with a nuclear membrane and organelles

L. Rate of deaths

M. Asexual reproduction in which the cell splits in half

FUNDAMENTAL CONCEPTS

14. Give an example of an organism that is normal flora and discuss what can occur if the organism is destroyed.

_____

_____

15. Using Table 7-1 in the text, list two health issues of concern in the 1990s.

_____

_____

16. List two characteristics of bacteria.

_____

_____

17. Explain the difference between a yeast fungus and a mold fungus.

_____

_____

18. List the three general types of bacterial shapes and give an example of each.

_____

_____

19. Match each bacterial shape or group with its name (see Figure 7-1 in the text).

_____   A. Bacilli

_____   B. Spirilla

_____   C. Streptococci

_____   D. Staphylococci

_____   E. Diplococci

20. Describe the benefits that flagella, spores, and capsules give to organisms that possess these structures.

_____

_____

_____

21. List four ways that a medical assistant can take precautions to prevent the spread of infection to others or to themselves.

_____

_____

22. When is the ideal time to collect a microbiology specimen?

_____

_____

23. Discuss the Jembec transport system.

_____

_____

24. Describe the cell wall structures that cause some organisms to be gram positive or gram negative.

_____

_____

25. Give the color of the gram-positive and gram-negative organisms after the decolorizer step has been applied.

_____

_____

26. Label the supplies needed for Gram's staining (see Procedure 7-2 in textbook).

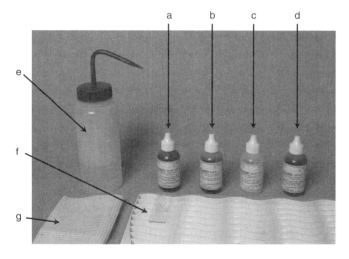

27. What is the causative agent for tuberculosis?

_____

_____

28. Describe the appearance and characteristics of *Trichomonas vaginalis*.

_____

_____

_____

29. Case study: On each blank below, write "C" if the statement is correct and "I" if the statement is incorrect. If the step is incorrect, explain why in the space provided.
    A medical assistant is performing Gram staining of a specimen.
    ___1. The specimen is heat fixed to fix the specimen to the slide.

    _____

    ___2. Crystal violet is applied to the slide for 2 minutes and then rinsed with water.

    _____

    ___3. Gram's iodine is applied for 1 minute and both gram-positive and gram-negative organisms are purple. Rinse with water.

    _____

    ___4. The decolorizer is applied until the purple has stopped running off the slide. This is the most critical step. Rinse with water.

    _____

    ___5. Safranin is applied last for 1 minute and rinsed with water. Gram-positive organisms are pink/red and gram-negative organisms are purple.

    _____

CLIA WAIVED MICROBIOLOGY TESTS

30. Describe the appearance of alpha, beta, and gamma hemolysis on blood agar plates.

_____

_____

_____

31. State the causative agent (genus and species) of strep throat and give the most common hemolytic reaction that this organism produces on blood agar plates.

_____

_____

_____

32. What antibiotic is in the disk that is used to identify *Streptococcus pyogenes*?

_____

33. Label the supplies needed to perform a Group A Streptococcus test (see Procedure 7-5 in textbook).

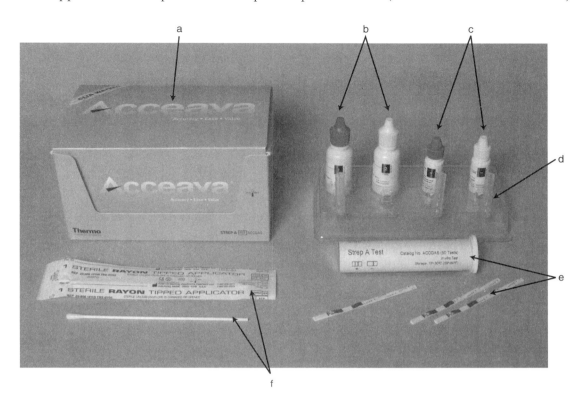

34. List three medical conditions associated with a strep infection.

_____

_____

_____

35. When discussing influenza, what is the difference between antigenic "drift" and "shift"?

_____

_____

_____

36. Label the supplies needed to perform an influenza test (see Procedure 7-6 in textbook).

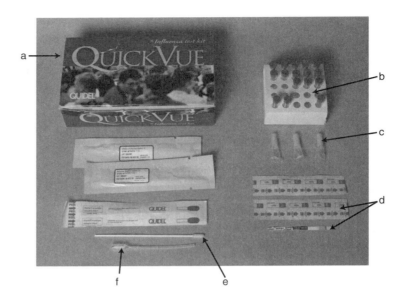

ADVANCED CONCEPTS

37. Give the oxygen requirements for aerobe, anaerobic, and facultative anaerobe organisms.

_____

_____

38. Name media requirements that most bacteria need for growth.

_____

_____

39. Explain how MacConkey media is a selective and a differential media.

_____

_____

40. Describe the shape, arrangement, and Gram stain appearance of *Neisseria gonorrhoeae*.

_____

41. Give the advantages of using an incinerator instead of a Bunsen burner.

_____

_____

42. Describe the differences between quadrant streaking and colony count streaking.

_____

_____

43. Explain a physician's reason for ordering a sensitivity test.

_____

_____

44. List three organisms that frequently cause urinary tract infections.

_____

_____

45. Case Study: By using Tables 7-3 through 7-9 in the text, complete the following information:

Streptococcus pneumoniae
- Gram stain reaction: _____
- Disease: _____
- Transmission: _____
- Specimens: _____

Neisseria gonorrhoeae
- Gram stain reaction: _____
- Disease: _____
- Transmission: _____
- Specimens: _____

Chlamydia trachomatis
- Disease: _____
- Transmission: _____
- Specimens: _____

Enterobius vermicularis
- Transmission: _____
- Specimens/tests: _____

Urinary tract infections
- Organisms: _____
- Gram stain reaction: _____
- Transmission: _____
- Tests/specimen: _____

Food poisoning (most common cause in the United States)
- Organisms: _____
- Gram stain reaction: _____
- Transmission: _____
- Tests/specimen: _____

Skill Procedure: Performing a Gram Stain

Person evaluated _____   Date _____

Evaluated by _____   Score/grade _____

Outcome goal	Perform a Gram stain
Conditions	Supplies required: - Gloves, bibulous paper, water bottle, or running water - Gram staining reagents: crystal violet, Gram's iodine, decolorizer, safranin - Staining rack
Standards	Required time = 15 minutes Performance time = _____ Total possible points = _____ Points earned = _____ Accuracy = final slide will show gram-positive and gram-negative bacteria
Evaluation rubric codes: **S** = Satisfactory, meets standard **U** = Unsatisfactory, fails to meet standard	
NOTE: Steps marked with an * are critical to achieve required competency.	

Preparation	Scores S	Scores U
*1. Sanitized hands and applied gloves		
*2. Fixed specimen to the slide (using heat or methanol)		
Procedure	**S**	**U**
*3. Crystal violet was applied to the slide for 1 minute		
4. Rinsed slide with water		
*5. Gram's iodine was applied to the slide for 1 minute		
6. Rinsed slide with water		
*7. The decolorizer was poured on and off until no more purple came off. Then the slide was rinsed with water to stop the reaction.		
*8. Safranin was applied for 1 minute		
9. Rinsed slide with water		
10. Blotted the slide dry in absorbent bibulous paper		
Follow-up	**S**	**U**
*11. Proper disposal and disinfection		
- Disinfected test area and instruments according to OSHA guidelines		
- Disposed regulated medical waste into biohazard bags (i.e., gloves)		
- Sanitized hands		
Total Points per Column		

Skill Procedure: Collection of Throat Specimen

Person evaluated _____ Date _____

Evaluated by _____ Score/grade _____

Outcome goal	Perform throat specimen collection
Conditions	Supplies required: - Sterile swabs and tongue depressor - Personal protective equipment
Standards	Required time = 10 minutes Performance time = _____ Total possible points = _____ Points earned = _____

Evaluation rubric codes:
S = Satisfactory, meets standard   **U** = Unsatisfactory, fails to meet standard

NOTE: Steps marked with an ✱ are critical to achieve required competency.

Preparation	Scores	
	S	**U**
✱1. Identified patient and placed in proper position		
- Had patient state name		
- Confirmed identification with patient		
- Compared with requisition		

Procedure	Scores	
	S	**U**
✱2. Sanitized hands and put on gloves and face mask		
✱3. Aseptically removed the sterile Dacron swab (cotton swab may inhibit growth of bacteria) from the package, holding only the tip of the swab		
4. Had the patient sit with head back		
✱5. Used a sterile tongue depressor to hold down the tongue and had patient say "ahh"		
✱6. Rotated the swab on the back of throat in a circular motion or figure-of-eight pattern		
- Did not touch the teeth or back of the tongue because these areas have normal flora		
- Two swabs can be used at the same time: one for a rapid Strep test and one for a culture if needed		
7. Inserted swab into appropriate container for testing		

Follow-up	Scores	
	S	**U**
8. Determined if patient was feeling well before dismissing		
✱9. Proper documentation was completed on patient chart (see below)		
✱10. Proper disposal and disinfection		
- Disinfected test area and instruments according to OSHA guidelines		
- Disposed regulated medical waste into biohazard bags (i.e., gloves, tongue depressor)		
✱11. Sanitized hands		
Total Points per Column		

Patient name: _____

Patient Chart Entry: (Don't forget to include when, what, how, why, any additional information, and the signature of the person charting.)

_____

_____

Analytical Test: Rapid Strep—Acceava Rapid Strep Kit

Person evaluated _____   Date _____

Evaluated by _____   Score/grade _____

Outcome goal	Perform FDA-approved CLIA waived rapid strep test following the most current OSHA safety guidelines and applying the correct quality control

Conditions	Supplies required:
	- Acceava rapid strep kit containing:
	  - Reagent 1 and reagent 2
	  - Liquid controls, positive and negative
	  - Soft plastic testing tubes
	  - Test stick and its container
	- Sterile rayon swab taken from wrapper
	- Sterile tongue depressor
	- Gloves, face protection

Standards	Required time = 10 minutes Performance time = _____ Total possible points = _____ Points earned = _____
Evaluation rubric codes: **S** = Satisfactory, meets standard **U** = Unsatisfactory, fails to meet standard	
NOTE: Steps marked with an ✶ are critical to achieve required competency.	

Preparation: Preanalytical Phase	Scores	
	S	**U**
A. Test information		
- Kit or instrument method **Strep A Test**		
- Manufacturer **Acceava**		
- Proper storage (temperature, light, etc.) **room temperature**		
- Lot # of kit _____		
- Expiration date _____		
- Package insert or test flow chart available ____ yes ____ no		
B. Specimen information		
- Type of specimen **throat swab using swab from kit (do not use cotton swabs)**		
C. Personal protective equipment: **gloves, facemask during throat swab, and biohazard container**		
Procedure: Analytical Phase	Scores	
	S	**U**
D. Performed/observed qualitative quality control		
- External liquid controls: positive _____ negative _____		
- Internal control: _____ (will appear as a red line on test stick)		
E. Performed patient test	**S**	**U**
1. Sanitized hands and applied gloves		
2. Just before testing, added three drops of reagent 1 and three drops of reagent 2 into the test tube. The solution should turn light yellow.		
3. Immediately put the throat swab into the extract solution		
4. Vigorously mixed the solution by rotating the swab forcefully against the side of the tube at least 10 times. Best results are obtained when the specimen is vigorously extracted in the solution.		

	S	U
5. Let stand for 1 minute, then squeeze the swab with the sides of the tube as the swab is withdrawn. Discarded the swab into a biohazard container.		
6. Removed a test stick from the container and recapped immediately. Placed the absorbent end of the test stick into the extracted sample in the tube.		
7. At 5 minutes read and recorded the results		
- Positive = a blue line in test area and pink line in control area indicating the internal control worked		
- Negative = no blue line in the test area and a pink line in control area indicating the internal control worked		

*Accurate Results _____ Instructor Confirmation _____

Follow-up/Postanalytical Phase	Scores	
	S	U
*F. Proper documentation		
1. On control/patient log _____ yes _____ no		
2. Documented on patient chart (see below)		
3. Identified critical values and took appropriate steps to notify physician		
- Expected values for analyte: negative for strep		
G. Proper disposal and disinfection		
1. Disposed all sharps into biohazard sharps containers		
2. Disposed all other regulated medical waste into biohazard bags		
3. Disinfected test area and instruments according to OSHA guidelines		
4. Sanitized hands after removing gloves		
Total Points per Column		

Patient name: _____

Patient Chart Entry: (Don't forget to include when, what, how, why, any additional information, and the signature of the person charting.)

_____

_____

_____

Analytical Test: Influenza—QuickVue Test Kit Method

Person evaluated _____   Date _____

Evaluated by _____   Score/grade _____

Outcome goal	Perform FDA-approved CLIA waived influenza test following the most current OSHA safety guidelines and applying the correct quality control
Conditions	Supplies required: QuickVue Test Kit containing: - Plastic tubes with buffer solution - Vials with extraction reagent solution - Individually packaged test strips - Positive control swab (provided in kit) - Patient soft foam nasal swab (or nasal wash equipment)
Standards	Required time = 10 minutes Performance time = _____ Total possible points = _____ Points earned = _____

Evaluation rubric codes:
S = Satisfactory, meets standard   **U** = Unsatisfactory, fails to meet standard

NOTE: Steps marked with an ✱ are critical to achieve required competency.

Preparation: Preanalytical Phase	Scores	
	S	U
A. Test information		
- Kit or instrument method **QuickVue Influenza Test A and B**		
- Manufacturer **Quidel**		
- Proper storage (temperature, light, etc.) **room temperature**		
- Lot # of kit _____		
- Expiration date _____		
- Package insert or test flow chart available _____ yes _____ no		
B. Specimen information		
- Type of specimen: **nasal swab using swab from kit or nasal wash**		
C. Personal protective equipment: gloves, facemask during nasal swab		

Procedure: Analytical Phase	Scores	
	S	U
D. Performed/observed qualitative quality control		
- External liquid controls: positive _____ negative _____		
- Internal control will appear as a blue line on test stick		
E. Performed patient test	S	U
1. Sanitized hands and applied gloves		
2. Dispensed all the reagent solution from the vial into the plastic tube containing buffer		
3. Added and swirled the nasal swab specimen in the solution, pressing against the sides of the tube to extract the specimen into the solution		
4. Removed the swab while pressing and rotating the swab against the tube to squeeze the liquid out of the swab		
5. Dipped the influenza test strip into the extraction solution		
6. Allowed 10 minutes for migration of the solution across the test area and control area of the strip and for the development of the results		

		Scores	
7. Test results for QuickVue A and B			
- Positive = a pink line in test area and blue line in control area indicating the internal control worked			
- Negative = no pink line in the test area and a blue line in the control area indicating the internal control worked.			
*Accurate Results _____ Instructor Confirmation _____			

Follow-up/Postanalytical Phase	S	U
*F. Proper documentation		
1. On control/patient log _____ yes _____ no		
2. Documentation on patient chart (see below)		
3. Identified critical values and took appropriate steps to notify physician		
- Expected values for analyte: negative for influenza A and B		
G. Proper disposal and disinfection		
1. Disposed all sharps into biohazard sharps containers		
2. Disposed all other regulated medical waste into biohazard bags		
3. Disinfected test area and instruments according to OSHA guidelines		
4. Sanitized hands after removing gloves		
Total Points per Column		

Patient name: _____

Patient Chart Entry: (Don't forget to include when, what, how, why, any additional information, and the signature of the person charting.)

_____

_____

_____

Appendix

Contents

LABORATORY RESPONSIBILITIES AND MAINTENANCE

FULL NAME OF TECH.	OFFICIAL INITIALS	TEMP CHECK DATE	DISINFECTED COUNTERS	OTHER

REFRIGERATOR/ROOM TEMPERATURE RECORD

REFRIGERATOR # _____   LOCATION _____

Refrigerator				Room		
Date	Temp	Tech		Date	Temp	Tech
----	----	----		----	----	----
____	____	____		____	____	____
____	____	____		____	____	____
____	____	____		____	____	____
____	____	____		____	____	____
____	____	____		____	____	____
____	____	____		____	____	____
____	____	____		____	____	____
____	____	____		____	____	____
____	____	____		____	____	____
____	____	____		____	____	____
____	____	____		____	____	____
____	____	____		____	____	____
____	____	____		____	____	____

Refrigerator acceptable range: Room acceptable range:
2° − 8° C. (+/− 1° C)   15° − 30° C (+/− 1° C)

Report discrepancies to your supervisor.

Unscheduled maintenance and repairs

_____
_____
_____
_____
_____
_____
_____
_____
_____
_____

URINE DIPSTICK QUALITY CONTROL LOG

DATE_____ URINE DIPSTICK CONTROL LEVEL _____ LOT #_____ EXPIRATION DATE_____

DATE	Reagent Strip Lot# Patient	DIPSTICK TESTS										CONFIRMATORY TESTS						ADD. TESTS		
		Leukocytes	Nitrites	Urobilinogen	Protein	pH	Blood	Specific Gravity	Ketones	Bilirubin	Glucose	Protein Method/Lot #	Ketones Method/Lot #	Glucose Method/Lot #	Bilirubin Method/Lot #	hCG Method/Lot #	Specific Gravity Refractometer	INITIAL

(From Zakus SM: *Clinical skills for medical assistants*, ed 4, St. Louis, 2001, Mosby.)

URINE DIPSTICK PATIENT LOG

DATE	Reagent Strip — Lot# — Patient	Leukocytes	Nitrites	Urobilinogen	Protein	pH	Blood	Specific Gravity	Ketones	Bilirubin	Glucose	Protein	Method/Lot #	Ketones	Method/Lot #	Glucose	Method/Lot #	Bilirubin	Method/Lot #	hCG	Method/Lot #	Specific Gravity Refractometer	INITIAL

DIPSTICK TESTS — *CONFIRMATORY TESTS* — *ADD. TESTS*

(From Zakus SM: *Clinical skills for medical assistants*, ed 4, St. Louis, 2001, Mosby.)

Quality Control   Flow Chart for HemoCue

Regardless of the purpose, most clinical testing procedures have the same quality control requirements. If an instrument is used, there is usually a method to check its mechanical function. Often this is nothing more than an 'optic check' or calibration strip supplied with the instrument to allow the user to determine whether the instrument is functional.

After determining that the instrument does indeed function, one then needs to prove that the reagents will perform as expected. Commonly, one uses a high and low value control sample. Look at the results. Are they within their expected ranges? If so, you can begin to test patients. If not, then it is time to do some troubleshooting.

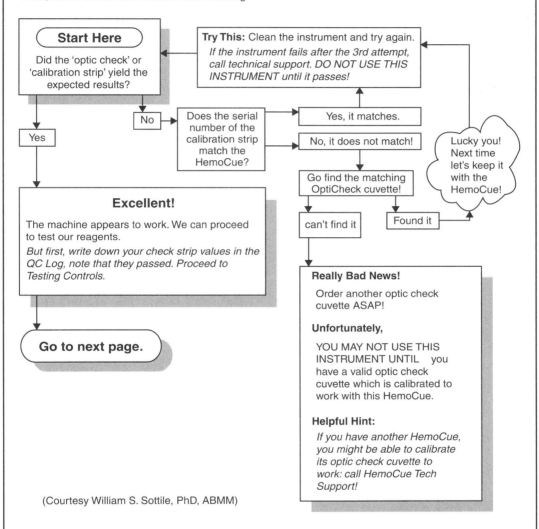

(Courtesy William S. Sottile, PhD, ABMM)

GENERIC QUANTITATIVE TEST CONTROL LOG (Template)

CONTROL LOT # _____   **EXPIRATION DATE** _____

CONTROL RANGE: _____   **CONTROL LEVEL** = _____

DATE	TECH	RESULT	ACCEPT	REJECT	CORRECTIVE ACTION

Generic Quantitative Test Procedure – Template

Quantitative Test _____

Person evaluated _____   Date _____

Evaluated by _____   Score/Grade _____

Outcome goal:	
Conditions:	
Standards:	Required Time = _____ minutes Performance Time = _____
	Total possible points = _____ Points earned = _____
Evaluation Rubric Codes:	
S = Satisfactory - Meets standard U = Unsatisfactory - Fails to meet standard	
NOTE: Steps marked with an * are critical to achieve required competency.	

Preparation – Preanalytical	Scores	
	S	U
A. Test Information		
- kit or instrumental method _____		
- Manufacturer _____		
- Proper storage (temp, light, etc.) _____		
- Lot number of kit or supplies _____		
- Expiration date _____		
- package insert and/or test flow chart available: _____ yes no _____		
B. Specimen Information		
- type of specimen and its preparation (i.e. fasting, first morning, etc.) _____		
- specimen container or testing device _____		
- amount of specimen _____		
C. Personal protective equipment _____		
D. Assembled all the above, sanitized hands, and applied PPE		

Procedure – Analytical Phase	Scores	
	S	U
E. Performed/Observed Quality Control for A. or B. below		
Quantitative testing controls		
- Calibration check _____		
- Control levels: Normal _____ High _____ Low _____		
F. Performed patient test: Followed proper steps (see flow chart and list steps)	S	U
1.		
2.		
3.		
4.		
5.		
6.		

	7.		
	8.		
	9.		
	10.		

＊Accurate Results _____   Instructor Confirmation _____

Follow-up / Post Analytical	Scores	
	S	U
＊ G. Proper Documentation		
1. On control log _____ yes _____ no		
2. On patient log _____ yes _____ no		
3. Documentation on patient chart – See below		
4. Identified "critical values" and took appropriate steps to notify physician EXPECTED VALUES FOR ANALYTE:		
H. Proper disposal and disinfection		
1. Dispose all sharps into biohazard sharps containers		
2. Dispose all other regulated medical waste into biohazard bags		
3. Disinfect test area and instruments according to OSHA guidelines		
4. Sanitize hands after removing gloves		
Column Totals =		

Patient Name: _____

Patient Chart Entry: (Don't forget to include when, what, how, why, any additional information, and the signature of the person charting.)

_____

_____

_____

HEMOGLOBIN QUALITY CONTROL LOG

TEST: _____   CONTROL LOT # _____

CONTROL RANGE: _____   FOR   LOW/NORMAL/HIGH CONTROL

DATE	TECH	RESULT	ACCEPT	REJECT	CORRECTIVE ACTION

HEMOGLOBIN PATIENT LOG

TEST: _____   KIT LOT # _____

Hemoglobin expected values =   Adult Males   = 13.0 – 18 g/dL
                                       Adult Females = 11.0 – 16.0 g/dL
                                       Infants   = 10.0 – 14.0 g/dL
                                       Children   = Increase to adult

DATE	TECH	PATIENT I.D.	RESULT	CHARTED

HEMATOCRIT QUALITY CONTROL LOG

TEST: _____   CONTROL LOT # _____

CONTROL RANGE: _____   FOR   LOW / NORMAL / HIGH CONTROL

DATE	TECH	SLOT #	RESULT	ACCEPT	REJECT	CORRECTIVE ACTION

HEMATOCRIT PATIENT LOG

Hematocrit expected values :

Adult Males = 42 – 52%
Adult Females = 36 – 48%
Infants = 32 – 38%
Children = Increase to adult

DATE	TECH	PATIENT I.D.	SLOT #	RESULT	CHARTED

ERYTHROCYTE SEDIMENTATION RATE PATIENT LOG

ESR expected values :

Adult Males < 50 years   = 0 – 15 mm/hr
Adult Males > 50 years   = 0 – 20 mm/hr
Adult Females < 50 years = 0 – 20 mm/hr
Adult Females > 50 years = 0 – 30 mm/hr

DATE	TECH	PATIENT I.D.	SLOT #	TIME	RESULT	CHARTED

PROTIME PATIENT LOG

ProTime expected values for both normal and therapeutic whole blood:

	INR	PT seconds (ISI = 1.0)
Normal	0.8 – 1.2	10.4 – 15.7 sec
Low anticoagulation	1.5 – 2.0	19.6 – 26.1 sec
Moderate anticoagulation	2.0 – 3.0	26.1 – 39.2 sec
High anticoagulation	2.5 – 4.0	32.6 – 52.2 sec

DATE	TECH	PATIENT I.D.	INR	PT seconds	CHARTED

GLUCOSE TEST CONTROL LOG

CONTROL LOT # _____   EXPIRATION DATE _____

CONTROL RANGE: _____   LEVEL: LOW/ NORMAL/ HIGH

DATE	TECH	RESULT	ACCEPT	REJECT	CORRECTIVE ACTION

GLUCOSE
PATIENT LOG

DATE	PATIENT	RESULT	CHARTED	TECH

HEMOGLOBIN A1c
PATIENT LOG

DATE	PATIENT	RESULT	CHARTED	TECH

CHOLESTECH LDX PATIENT LOG

_____

Cassette Lot #: _____ Expiration Date: _____ LDX Serial #: _____

Date	Operator	Patient I.D.	Charted	TRG	TC	GLU	HDL	LDL	TC/HDL	ALT

HEMOCCULT
PATIENT LOG

DATE	PATIENT	RESULT	TECH

QUALITATIVE CONTROL AND PATIENT LOG (TEMPLATE)

TEST: _____

KIT NAME AND MANUFACTURER: _____

LOT#:_____   EXPIRATION DATE: _____

STORAGE REQUIREMENTS:_____   TEST FLOW CHART: _____

DATE	SPECIMEN I.D. (CONTROL/PATIENT)	RESULT (+ OR −)	INTERNAL CONTROL PASSED (Y or N)	CHARTED IN PATIENT RECORD	TECH INITIALS

Generic Qualitative Test Procedure – Template

Qualitative Test _____

Person evaluated _____   Date _____

Evaluated by _____   Score/Grade _____

Outcome goal:	
Conditions:	Supplies required:
Standards:	Required Time = _____ minutes Performance Time = _____
	Total possible points = _____ Points earned = _____

Evaluation Rubric Codes:

S = Satisfactory - Meets standard   U = Unsatisfactory - Fails to meet standard

NOTE: Steps marked with an * are critical to achieve required competency.

Preparation – Preanalytical	Scores	
	S	U
A. Test Information		
- kit method		
- Manufacturer		
- Proper storage (temp, light, etc.)		
- Lot number of kit _____		
- Expiration date _____		
- package insert and/or test flow chart available: _____ yes _____ no		
B. Personal protective equipment		
C. Specimen Information		

Procedure – Analytical Phase	Scores	
	S	U
D. Performed/Observed Qualitative Quality Control		
- External liquid controls: Positive _____ Negative _____		
- Internal control:		
E. Performed patient test	S	U
1.		
2.		

3.			
4.			
POSITIVE seen as:			
NEGATIVE seen as:			
INVALID seen as:			
*Accurate Results _____ Instructor Confirmation _____			

	Scores	
Follow-up / Post Analytical	**S**	**U**
✳ F. Proper documentation		
1. On control/patient log _____ yes _____ no		
2. Documentation on patient chart – See below		
3. Identified "critical values" and took appropriate steps to notify physician EXPECTED VALUES FOR ANALYTE:		
G. Proper disposal and disinfection		
1. Disposed all sharps into biohazard sharps containers		
2. Disposed all other regulated medical waste into biohazard bags		
3. Disinfected test area and instruments according to OSHA guidelines		
4. Sanitized hands after removing gloves		
Column Totals =		

Patient Name: _____

Patient Chart Entry: (Don't forget to include when, what, how, why, any additional information, and the signature of the person charting.)

_____

_____

_____

HEALTH ASSESSMENT FORM

Please print clearly:

Date _____

Name _____ Address _____

City _____ State _____ ZIP _____

Telephone _____ Age (date of birth) ____/____/____ Sex _____ Race _____

Ht. _____ Wt. _____

Do you consider yourself overweight? _____ If so, how much? _____

Name of family Doctor _____ When last seen? _____

Do you smoke? _____ If yes, how many packs a day _____ Alcohol use? _____

Do you have :   _____ Heart Trouble   _____ High Blood Pressure

                         _____ Kidney Problems   _____ Heart Attack Before / After 40

Are you taking medication for Cholesterol? _____ Blood Pressure? _____ Other? _____

Do you exercise regularly? _____ When did you last eat? _____ hours

When you are finished with all your tests, please return to this room or your instructor for final review of your results.

RELEASE:

I RELEASE _____ and the _____ Students from any
liability as a result of my participation in this Health Fair.

Signature _____ Date _____

Parent/Guardian _____ Witness _____ **REFERENCE #** _____

TEST	NORMAL LIMITS	RESULTS	FURTHER EVALUATION _____

URINALYSIS

Glucose	NEG
Bilirubin	NEG
Ketone	NEG
Spec Grav	1.005 – 1.030
Blood	NEG
pH	6.0 – 8.0
Protein	NEG/TRACE
Urobil.	NORM
Nitrite	NEG
Leukocytes	NEG

Clinitek * indicates further evaluation

Urinalysis

Routine urinalysis is a basic test, but it provides the physician with a tremendous amount of information when a disease process is present. This test can help confirm or rule out a suspected diagnosis. It is a routine test repeated annually or as frequently as necessary to evaluate the patient's health status.

HEMATOLOGY

ANEMIA   Hemoglobin: greater than 12 mg/dl.   _____

Hematocrit: greater than 32%   _____

Anemia Check

The hemoglobin and hematocrit tests determine the oxygen-carrying ability of the blood. They are simple and efficient methods to detect any <u>anemia</u>. A patient is considered anemic if the hemoglobin value is below 12 mg/dl, or the hematocrit is below 34%. Low values are caused by hemorrhage, pregnancy, recent menstruation, iron deficiency, or other causes which the physician would need to evaluate.

ESR Erythrocyte Sedimentation Rate = 0 – 20 mm/hr _____

Erythrocyte sedimentation rates are increased in infections and inflammatory diseases, tissue destruction, and other conditions that lead to an increase in plasma fibrinogen.

REFERENCE # _____

TEST	NORMAL LIMITS	RESULTS	FURTHER EVALUATION _____

QBC – Complete Blood Count

QBC Reference Ranges		
Hematocrit Males (%)	42.0 – 50.0	--------------
Hematocrit Females (%)	36.0 – 45.0	--------------
Hemoglobin Males (g/dL)	14.0 – 18.0	--------------
Hemoglobin Females (g/dL)	12.0 – 16.0	--------------
MCHC (g/dL)	31.7 – 36.0	--------------
Platelet Count (x10^9/L)	140 – 440	--------------
WBC (x10^9/L)	4.3 – 10.0	--------------
Granulocyte Count (x10^9/L)	1.8 – 7.2	--------------
Lymphocyte/Monocyte Count (x10^9/L)	1.7 – 4.9	--------------

COAGULATION

ProTime-3

results _____ INR
_____ seconds

Desirable 0.8 – 1.2 INR
10.4 – 15.7 seconds
Therapeutic 1.5 – 4.0 INR

BLOOD CHEMISTRY

GLUCOSE

Fasting _____ (8 or more hrs since eating)
-OR-
Random (# of hours since eating) _____ hrs.
Blood Sugars
Normal 80-125 (if 2 hrs after eating). Result = _____

WARNING SIGNS OF DIABETES	
TYPE I DIABETES	**TYPE II DIABETES**
Constant urination	Drowsiness
Abnormal thirst	Itching
Unusual hunger	A family history of diabetes
The rapid loss of weight	Blurred vision
Irritability	Excessive weight
Obvious weakness or fatigue	Tingling, numbness in feet
Nausea and vomiting	Easy fatigue
	Skin infections and slow healing

GLYCOSYLATED HEMOGLOBIN Desirable levels are below 7.

Result _____

REFERENCE #_____

TEST	NORMAL LIMITS	RESULTS	FURTHER EVALUATION _____

TOTAL CHOLESTEROL:

8 hr. **Fasting** preferred _____ **or Random** hours since eating _____ Results = _____ mg/dl   [ ]

        200 mg/dl or less   = Recommended
        200 – 239 mg/dl   = Border line to high risk
        240 mg/dl or above = High risk

Cholesterol

Cholesterol measurements are used in the diagnosis and monitoring of disorders involving excess cholesterol in the blood and of fat metabolism disorders. These conditions are often associated with coronary heart disease. It is believed that lowering the mean value of cholesterol levels will reduce coronary heart disease.

LIPID PROFILE: (CHOLESTECH TEST)   [ ]

Lipid Profile	Desirable Numbers:	Cholestech results
Total Cholesterol (TC)	less than 200 mg/dL	
HDL Cholesterol	greater than 40 mg/dL	
LDL Cholesterol	less than 130 mg/dL	
Triglycerides	less than 150 mg/dL	
TC/HDL Ratio	4.5 or less	
Glucose	fasting: 60-110 mg/dL	
	Nonfasting: less than 160 mg/dL	

FECAL OCCULT BLOOD   **Results (Positive or Negative)**

BLOOD TYPE   **ABO** _____   **Rh** _____

IMMUNOLOGY/MICROBIOLOGY TEST _____

        POSITIVE _____   **NEGATIVE** _____

                                                              REFERENCE # _____

PROFESSIONAL EVALUATION FORM
For LABORATORY CLASSROOM

STUDENT: _____ DATE: _____

CLASS: _____ SEMESTER: _____

NUMBER OF TARDIES: _____ NUMBER OF HOURS ABSENT: _____

CLASSROOM PROFESSIONALISM

OBJECTIVE	VERY SATISFACTORY 3	SATISFACTORY 2	UNSATISFACTORY 1	COMMENTS (See below)
Exhibits professional written communication (Appearance, language, grammar, etc.)				
Utilizes the class materials appropriately (Equipment, supplies, computers, clean-up, etc.)				
Provides instructor with all necessary information in a timely and organized manner (Meets due dates, make-ups turned in within a week, etc.)				
Adheres to specific course policies (Make-up guidelines, skill check-offs, externship guidelines, etc.)				
Projects a positive attitude and motivation (Seen during lectures and labs)				
Displays professional verbal communication at all times (Respectful, tactful, etc.)				
Maintains confidentiality of all personal interactions at all times (See rules of confidentiality in handbook)				
Projects professional work ethics (Responsible, accountable, independent, full use of lab time: practice, study, computer, etc.)				
Cooperates with fellow students (Team projects, skill practice, study groups)				
Displays responsible attendance behavior (Arriving on time, calling in if detained or absent, prepared for next class session)				
Dresses appropriately (see handbook)				

Comments: _____

_____

Student Signature _____ Instructor_____